WHAT ADVANC
ABOUT

MW01140679

"Throughout this story flows the undercurrent that is the healing power of nature. Pat has survived—and thrived—not only because of fantastic medical treatment, but also because of his ability to patch into this power. May you find your own power in these pages. It is a field guide to resiliency amid adversity."

-Alan Hobson,
Two-Time Cancer Survivor, Mt. Everest Climber & Summiteer
Author, *Climb Back from Cancer*
Creator, the Climb Back from Cancer Survivorship Program

"In a friendship that has spanned six decades, I have seen firsthand on many occasions Pat Herzog's passion and love for nature. This book captures the important story of how nature helped him heal and reclaim his life. As we paddled, hiked and explored together in the months and years after he faced off with cancer, I was impressed by his toughness and tenacity. For this I call him Wolf."

-Bill Berry,
Author, *Banning DDT, How Citizen Activists in Wisconsin Led the Way*

"Pat Herzog and I grew up in similar circumstances, though 600 miles apart, before our life streams converged at Delta, Manitoba in 1972. The sense of awe and excitement that Pat describes at his accelerating understanding of nature resonates deeply with me. Wetlands like Delta are wondrous and vibrant places that merit our study and care. As Pat met and eventually overcame his illness, nature clearly offered a vital touchstone— something that mattered even more than his illness."

-Michael G. Anderson, Ph.D., Emeritus Scientist
Ducks Unlimited Canada

"Pat Herzog weaves his love of nature throughout this powerful, honest and touching story of sorrow and uplift as he unrelentingly faces the scourge of cancer and its treatments. From a harrowing bone marrow transplant through physical and mental pain and severe debilitating fatigue Pat emerges whole through his lifelong connection with the restorative/curative/spiritual power of nature."

-Dr. Linda E. Carlson, Ph.D., C.Psych.
Professor Department of Oncology
University of Calgary

Clinical Psychologist and Director of Research
Department of Psychosocial Resources
Tom Baker Cancer Centre

"In *From the Mist*, Pat Herzog takes us on a both harrowing and enlightening journey with his bout with cancer. Although modern medicine can do wonders, Pat demonstrates there is more to the healing process: the omnipotent restorative energy of nature—a powerful and readily available resource. A must-read for anyone facing serious illness, this book offers more than just hope. Pat shares his path from the dark mist of illness into the healing light."

-Rob Kaye,
Author, *Born to the Wild: Journals of a National Park Warden in the Canadian Rockies*

"I loved this book! The nature daydreams, woven throughout the battle with cancer, reinforced my own beliefs in healing. Pat's heartwarming honesty of the seemingly insurmountable challenges of this disease, and his stepwise accounts of recovery guided by nature, is simply good medicine for us all."

-Tim Clermont
Conservation Land and Habitat Securement Manager
The Nature Trust of British Columbia

From The Mist

A LIFE RESTORED BY NATURE

by Patrick Walter Herzog

From The Mist
Copyright © 2017 by Patrick Walter Herzog
First Edition — 2017

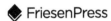 FriesenPress

Suite 300 - 990 Fort St
Victoria, BC, V8V 3K2
Canada

www.friesenpress.com

Cover Image: Twilight - Siberian Tiger by Robert Bateman.

Images Copyright © Robert Bateman. All rights reserved.
www.batemancentre.org

Owing to limitations of space, permissions to reprint previously published material appear on pages 174-176.

Paper: FSC certified

ISBN
978-1-4602-9271-6 (Hardcover)
978-1-4602-9272-3 (Paperback)
978-1-4602-9273-0 (eBook)

1. NATURE

2. HEALTH & FITNESS, HEALING

3. HEALTH & FITNESS, DISEASES, CANCER

Distributed to the trade by The Ingram Book Company

For Kathy, of course,
who upon hearing my voice on the phone will ask,
"What part of me do you want today?"

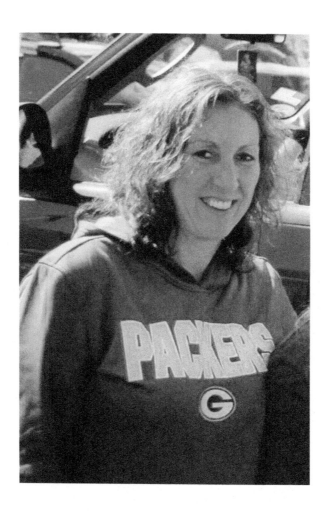

Contents

PART III — DRY GROUND

Author's Note

I wrote this book because nature saved my life.

I did not climb a mountain to obtain self-enlightenment. I did not hike across the wilderness to banish my demons. I did not sail across an ocean to test my mettle. The cancer I had was in complete remission, but I was dying anyway, until I was rescued by nature.

Perhaps this is not surprising, because nature has always been my companion.

It was waiting outside the back door when houses like ours were invading the rural countryside that was Green Bay, Wisconsin in the 1950s. Honeybees and bumblebees swarmed through neighborhood lawns overrun with white clover and dandelion—my friends and I caught them in glass mayo jars, pounding nail holes into the lids so the insects could breathe. We chased monarch butterflies, and the rarer yellow swallowtails, and at dusk we watched bats dive at the green apples we threw into the sky, telling the youngest among us that bats could get snarled in their hair. We looked for fireflies in hay meadows, and toads in window wells under the streetlights.

We had secret camps in the nearby parcels of vacant forest— stands of oak, maple, basswood and hickory. We reached them by sneaking through the orchard that bounded our neighborhood, crawling through the culverts underneath the railroad tracks we were forbidden to cross, and running across pastures, ducking beneath electric fences to escape the curious dairy cows that followed (and scared) us.

We built forts, stuck our hands in anthills as a test of strength, lit stick matches on the zippers of our pants, ate burned hot dogs off the ends of sharpened sticks, and learned to avoid stinging nettles and poison ivy. I pretended to be Daniel Boone

When cancer crept in decades later, I was somewhere in the jungles of Costa Rica.

This is the story of how I was renewed by nature.

Most of the writing was done from a cliff on Vancouver Island while I looked across the vast distance of the Salish Sea past the dark outline of Texada Island to the snowy peaks of mainland British Columbia. Towering Douglas firs and western hemlocks bounded my view, and bracken fern, thimbleberry, and maple saplings tumbled downhill for more than a hundred winding steps before mixing along the shore with thickets of salal. An oyster bed lay in the rocky shallows just offshore.

Some days the gentle waves were whipped into whitecaps, catching the miles of wind I could not see. Whatever the weather, it was a good place, whether I was inside or out, to contemplate my life before and after cancer.

My primary companions were the birds outside my big windows. Dark-eyed juncos darted around the yard year-round, while spotted towhees scratched beneath the brush until winter. If I brought their feeders inside at night, Anna's hummingbirds stayed despite the occasional subfreezing days. The cold weather brought varied thrushes—deep-forest "robins" with exotic markings—to replace the robins that usually sprinted across the grass. I never saw them together.

Most days I was happily distracted by the bald eagles that claimed ownership of the lone fir tree rising above the slope, forever scolding the crows trying to share its weathered crown of branches. The tree, a titan of the temperate rainforest, is twenty-five stories high and rivals the girth and height of the giants of the canopy I remember from my studies in the tropical forests of Costa Rica.

I had to resist the desire to be sitting quietly outdoors, watching and hearing the birds. Often that task was daunting, especially on days when my mind started to whirl aimlessly as I forced myself to hen-peck for letters on the keyboard. Some effects of treatment still linger—science now knows why, but that is another story.

My message is simple: nature heals. It always has. Mind, body, and spirit. Heart and soul.

Now get outside and open your senses.

Pat Herzog
Qualicum Beach, B.C.
September 2017

Prologue

Nature, from the Latin, *nasci*, to "be born."

The path downhill through the winter-flattened grass was a bit wider, and the brush was slightly thicker in the little woods above the cancer centre. The poplar trees looked the same, however, their growth forever stunted by the chinook winds that roar through them. I paused to watch and listen for wood-peckers as I had once done clad in my hospital gown.

Nothing much seemed to have changed on Unit 57, either. Dr. Chaudhry was parked at a workstation, the same one where I had last seen him—charts on his lap, patient data on a computer screen, a nurse hovering alongside.

I waited nearby for a quiet moment before catching his eye. He returned my greeting with a solid handshake, and warm eyes I would never forget.

"You are looking well, Mr. Herzog," he said, "wonderful to see you again."

"Thank you, doctor. You too. I hope you're not working too hard," I said (knowing full well the massive number of hours he logged every week).

"What brings you by?"

"I'm posting my photo for this year on the bulletin board. Bolek (the man who ensures the unit runs smoothly day *and* night) makes certain I don't forget."

As per tradition, I am outside during the first week of February, in a swimsuit, wherever I am, holding a small sign denoting the year. Bolek says I fooled everyone the time I posed at home in the sun standing beneath a beach umbrella— no one could believe the whitest sand they had ever seen was indeed snow. He tells me my willingness to stand barefoot, and bare-chested, outside during winter, inspires both patients and staff almost as much as my steady run of pictures (seventeen years and counting).

Usually I would sneak in and leave without talking to anyone, anxious to be unnoticed, but today I have something to ask Dr. Chaudhry.

"You know, if there is anything I can ever do for you, just let me know."

He smiles happily, mischievously and says, "You already let us kick the crap out of you, you don't have to do anything else."

He has yet to learn I am writing a book about my journey with cancer. And why without nature by my side he would not be seeing me today.

PART I
BUSHWHACKED

I wish I could have him in my clinic. He is a truly nice person with an interesting disease that he will need to endure.

–Thomas J. Saphner, M.D., Medical Oncologist, St. Vincent's Hospital, Green Bay, Wisconsin

Chapter 1
Endangered

It is one thing to see, and especially to hear, a scarlet macaw in a home or zoo.

It is quite another thing to observe them in the wild.

–Robert Bateman, artist/naturalist

I awake in the steamy darkness, reaching for the pop-up travel alarm. I stuff it under the pillow, not moving again until the park guards resume their snoring. Daybreak is two hours away yet it is time to go.

A mosquito net drapes my bunk, and I think of old Tarzan movies while wiggling into my pants and shirt. I slip beneath the mesh and grab my boots, shaking them upside down (occasionally a scorpion drops out). Sliding in stocking feet across the creaking floor, I stop whenever I hear the rustle of sheets. A mouse scampers into the shadows.

My pack hangs by the back door, safe from the hungry mice. The building sits on stilts, and the pesky creatures (along with rats) feed on the loose rice and beans that drop through the wide cracks in the kitchen floor.

The rodents are a problem; they attract the fearsome fer-de-lance or *terciopelo*, the most aggressive pit viper in Costa Rica. These night-hunting snakes often hide near the bunkhouse, waiting to ambush their prey. Broom in hand, I peer out the screen door, ready to sweep the porch and steps clear of danger—a misstep near these big snakes (up to seven feet long) is almost certain to cause a devastating, venom-laden strike. Warning shots are rare.

The jungle is a dark presence that closes around me as I pedal away from the station. And when something thumps and hits the forest floor, silencing the ragged chorus of countless night insects, the boy in me still imagines something big out there—deliberately and furtively on the move—rather than a tree limb finally overcome by its burden of mosses and epiphytes.

Pedaling is faster than walking, despite the wicked potholes that litter the road, and the discomfort of sitting on a skinny banana seat with my knees near my chin (somehow the guards patrol in tandem). I abandon the bike at a path that I constantly reclaim from a chaotic foliage of creeping vines and clutching plants of a hundred different sizes, shapes, and colors of green. Some of the smaller palms are armed with stout black needles.

I now have an hour on foot to reach my destination. My eyes strain to see beyond the arc of my searchlight: I want to hurry, afraid of losing time, the sky black beneath the trees. I routinely remove the large debris that continually falls on the trail, but I go slowly. Any fine details I fail to see on the jungle floor could shift my walk from benign to deadly: the snakebite serum I carry is not a cure, and the park guards only have a vague notion of my route (and they are still asleep).

The trail slides outside the park to the floodplain of the Tárcoles River. Here the pampas grass is over my head and strung with spider webs. Some of the clinging arachnids have bi-colored legs that easily extend beyond the edges of standard dinner plates. Similar spiders hang from the eaves of our house in San Rafael, and my young girls hunt them at night with flashlights.

I arrive at a steep hill. I do not like climbing through the slick grass that incessantly defies my efforts to cut it, because if I slip, my bare hands touch the ground (and whatever lives there). The top of the rise, however, is the only place from where I can accurately count the flock of scarlet macaws that are still sleeping in the mangrove swamp a few miles away.

The birds are one of only two significant populations remaining in the country. Habitat destruction, poaching of nests, and illegal trade have decimated the numbers of these regal birds throughout Costa Rica, and my flock is in danger of extinction. Indeed, the macaws—revered by the Aztecs, Mayas and Incas—have been severely reduced in numbers throughout most of their formerly extensive range.

I wait in the dark, looking at the burning stars. In temperate areas, where I am used to being in the field, the darkest hours before dawn brighten slowly, the sky changing from black to gray, then purple, and finally a blue of some color. Here, after the first gray moments of the morning race away from the night, vapors of mist rise quickly above the green-black forest, and orange-yellow daylight strikes my back. Immediately, the shrieks of the macaws and the booming roars of howler monkeys pierce the pre-dawn stillness.

Cat-like screeches sweep toward me: the vanguard of birds is closing fast. I cannot see them flying through the river fog below me, but then a bright torrent of crimson, yellow, and blue crests the hill: a dozen macaws, lit by the rising sun. Gold metallic iridescence flashes beneath their wings as they dart and weave to avoid me, squawking amid a wild display of color and sound. The birds are one of the largest parrots in the world, nearly three feet long from their creamy faces to the end of pointed tails that are, incredibly, more than half of their length. Despite having been imprinted on nature's wonders as a child, I pinch myself to ensure the noisy spectacle is real.

I watch them fly—above me, beside me and below me—free and without bars. If I could only jump a little higher, reach a bit further, I could touch one. I almost forget to count them, still shaking my head in disbelief that I am truly here, surrounded by the raucous riot of flaming color. If the boa constrictor I saw earlier in the week was climbing my leg right now, I would not know it.

For ninety minutes, I tally the macaws that pass by, whether singles, or pairs calling to young birds in tow. Then all the birds are gone, streaking to the highlands to forage for fruit and nuts. Silence returns to the valley, with only the tilted wings of vultures aloft in the pale bright sky.

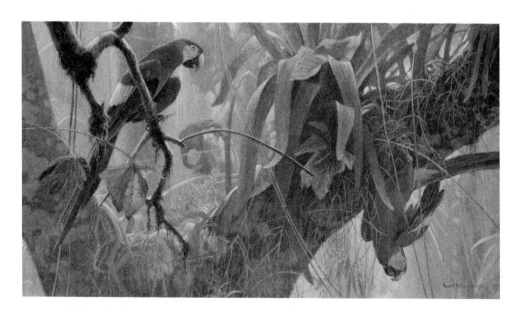

Tropical Canopy – Scarlet Macaws

I would like to linger, then go and watch the crocodiles along the river—maybe that big monster I saw last month will be there—but the cook is waiting to fry eggs and tortillas to go with my late breakfast of rice and beans. I hurry back to the bike, the daylight helping to clear the trail of danger. Legions of leaf-cutter ants carrying their oversized loads of forage now catch my eye.

I will repeat the survey again at dusk, when the macaws return to the mangroves. The guards tease me, saying I will get snatched by a jaguar one of these nights. Not by one of the big cats (which rarely attack humans), but by a *nagual,* a mystical and beautiful witch that takes the shape of an evil jaguar or puma. I will only notice one if I see a black shadow even darker than the surrounding night. Although I dismiss such foolishness, I pedal faster each evening when I see the distant glow of the guardhouse lights (or imagine the air closing too swiftly behind me).

Following a week of surveys, I return to our home near the campus of the National University of Costa Rica, where I have a position in the Program of Regional Studies in the Management of Wildlife. Besides determining the status of the macaws, and seeking protection for sea turtles, I teach field research techniques to master's degree students from countries in central and South America. The work has quickly become a major highlight of my decades-long career in wildlife conservation.

After two years, my sabbatical at an end, I record the flight of the macaws a final time. I worry about the fate of the birds: they need help. The population has continued to decline and they are classified as endangered, a species in immediate danger of extinction. I hope to return soon, anxious to help design a recovery plan that will ensure their survival.

Lately, however, I have been unusually tired after the morning counts, napping before lunch instead of practicing Spanish with the guards. We've been making extra trips to the beach before our departure, packing our stuff repeatedly for air travel, and unsuccessfully trying to say one final good-bye to our many *tico* friends. I blame the whirlwind of activity and the rush to finish my fieldwork for my persistent lack of energy, certain I will rebound after we arrive in Green Bay, Wisconsin, to spend Christmas with our parents before driving across the frozen prairies to our home in western Canada.

Chapter 2

The Northwoods

So woods are spooky . . . though you tell yourself it's preposterous, you can't quite shake the feeling that you are being watched.

–Bill Bryson, *A Walk in the Woods: Rediscovering America on the Appalachian Trail*

Our holiday visit to Wisconsin coincides with the ten-day deer hunt that traditionally occurs in late November during the week of Thanksgiving. My dad, who has gone deer hunting with the same seven friends continuously since before I was born, has missed the past two seasons, complaining of dizzy spells. My mom and I suspect, however, that the mysterious ailment is mainly an excuse to avoid the effort to get packed. He has agreed to head north if I organize our gear, and *if* I can be content to watch the woods while sitting together in the truck when he gets woozy (he knows my distaste for anything that resembles road hunting).

It is a rare opportunity—it has been twenty years since we sat in the woods side by side. The last time was the year before I left home to pursue my master's degree in wildlife biology in Canada.

As a boy, I slept with a deer head above my bed, dreaming of the day I would go to the mysterious Northwoods. I wanted to be a hunter too, and I would only eat my cooked carrots and peas when my mom deemed them "hunter food."

Every year, my dad would call home once from his hunting trip; I would hear his voice over the phone, crackling with long-distance and wilderness. Finally, when I was thirteen years old, I was old enough to join the other boys in camp.

★   ★   ★   ★   ★

The snow that was a dusting at home was a blizzard when I arrived at the bus station in Eagle River. Mountains of plowed snow tumbled into the streets, and the winding road to the deer camp—a clapboard cabin where I woke to bits of sifted snow on my blankets—was surrounded by miles of unbroken forest. I pasted my face to the window, watching for deer at every turn.

My dad carved my initials next to his own on a paper birch tree near a worn deer trail. We sat side-by-side on boat cushions, watching the forest together for a few days before I went alone before dawn, following the ghostly outlines of the trees to what was now my stand.

I could sit there for hours, listening for the crack of twigs, the crunch of leaves, or the dull pop of frozen snow. I learned to tell time without a watch, using the temperature of the chill air, shading in the trees, and the light in the sky to judge the passing of the day. Only my eyes moved as I scanned the forest—I ate my lunch in hurried bites.

After supper, I would dry my clothes, chop firewood and bucket water from holes I cut in the frozen lake. The work was no more than the wilderness life I had longed to live ever since I had read *Lost in the Barrens* by Farley Mowat. Then I would crawl into bed, hearing the laughter and chink of beer bottles around the card table, my mind replaying the scenes of the day until I fell asleep.

Deer were few—I rarely saw one. But I never got cold or bored, each moment rife with the anticipation of a huge whitetail buck threading his way through the trees toward my stand. And the biggest buck I had ever dreamed of appeared during that first year in the woods.

It was a cloudless day, the sunlight bouncing sharply off the fresh snow in a nearby opening (where a day earlier I had seen my first snowshoe hare). I was blinded by the glare, so I seldom looked that way, certain I would catch any movement with the corner of my eye.

Late afternoon, not a sound, the thick cedars both green and black. A long shaft of light in the clearing. And a buck, staring at me—magical, motionless—with antlers that seemed impossibly huge and real.

I must have blinked because suddenly the buck was gone—without movement, without sound.

When it was dusk I walked to the spot, needing proof of our brief encounter. There were tracks, but not many, and I could not tell which way he had gone.

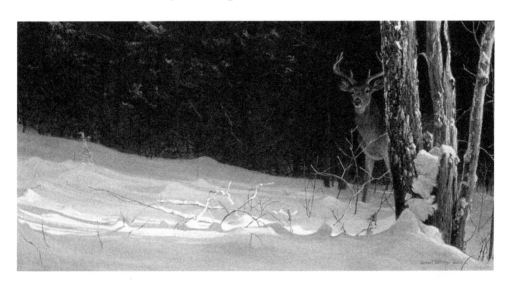

Whitetail in Winter

Patrick Walter Herzog

I liked being on my own in the woods, wild country around me. Black-capped chickadees and whiskey jacks (gray jays) often landed a few feet away from me, occasionally standing on my boot or knee. Grouse and squirrels passed by, unaware I was intrigued by their every behavior.

The veteran hunters warned me, however, that animals with fangs and claws—*predators*—were also in the woods. Especially ornery black bears looking for places to hibernate.

I was afraid of bears. They were always frothing at the mouth, snapping their teeth, and raising their claws on the covers of my dad's *Outdoor Life* magazines. And when I picked blackberries with Dad in the summer, yelling and banging my metal pails together to shoo bears away (as I was told), he would scare me by growling from the other side of the patch.

The men said I should not only be wary of coyotes, foxes, and bobcats, but that I should shoot them, or any other critter with fur or feathers that might pose a threat to deer (or rabbits). When I did see a bobcat, however, picking his way through the forest, rubbing his face on branches, scratching his ears, and sniffing the snow, he did not seem dangerous to me.

But what about wolves? I was told they were the scourge of the Northwoods, hunting in packs, killing deer, but eating few. One of the men swore he had seen their massive tracks the previous year. Dad said if I ever saw them, I should climb a tree and yell for him.

I thought he was likely teasing—the stories I had read said it was a myth that wolves attacked people. The wolf report in the big-game hunting regulations indicated that after being shot, trapped, and poisoned ruthlessly for years, wolves had likely disappeared from *most* of the state.

One day, after staying late on my stand, I was hurrying through the dark forest to reach the open ridge that led back to camp. When I stepped into the blue twilight, I stopped in mid-stride.

Somewhere ahead, on the edge of the bush, I felt there was something watching me.

Was it wolves? It must be wolves to jar my senses with such force.

I walked slowly. I knew they were there watching me, fading cautiously into the trees. I could not find their tracks the next day (it had snowed several inches overnight), but, as I was to learn many times in the years ahead, I would be foolish to dismiss such uncanny field experiences with wildlife as merely imaginary.

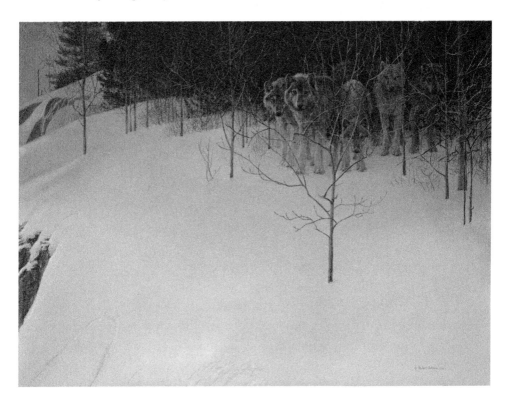

Clear Night – Wolves

★ ★ ★ ★ ★

The forest is buried in soft snow when we arrive at camp the day before hunting. I tell Dad I have brought along my sandals—he asks if I plan on running through the trees waving a machete.

I'm wearing a pair of his boots, however, while kicking a path through the snow to my old stand. When we examine the birch tree for our initials, only mine are vaguely visible. Dad asks me if I am still afraid of bears.

By the end of the next day, my heart pounds so loudly in my ears I cannot hear anything else, and I begin to feel something ominous invading my consciousness.

Nothing is wrong in the woods—if there was, I would know.

Yet my intuition insists there is a need to be wary, as if there is unseen danger, something abnormal. Whatever is unsettling me is impervious to the wonders of the winter forest I should be experiencing as I scan the trees for deer. I feel edgy and strangely overtired, and I forgo any long walks to see what is over the next hill, hoping that by resting I will regain my stamina and well-being. But by the end of the week I am still weak, and uneasiness overpowers any joy I feel about hunting

While drinking coffee with Dad, leaning on the tailgate of his truck during our last day in the field, I reluctantly share the concerns dogging my days and plaguing my final thoughts at night. I hesitate to worry him, unwilling to disturb the happiness I have seen in his eyes while enjoying the camaraderie of his old friends. Clayton, his best friend, has told me often how great it was for Dad to be back.

"Hey, Dad, I haven't been feeling very well. Maybe I brought back a bug from Costa Rica."

"I suppose it could be that, but you seem all right to me," he replies, taking a sip of coffee.

"Maybe it's the quick change to winter weather," I suggest, kicking snow by the tire.

"Whatever you think, Pat." Clapping me on the back, he adds, "I do know one thing."

"What's that, Dad?"

"You haven't been drinking your share of the beer this week."

Drinking beer hasn't mixed favorably with my recurring worries of somehow being unwell. Even playing cribbage with the old-timers (still for only a quarter a game) has lost its fun.

A few days after returning from hunting, my heart rate is racing so wildly I go to the emergency room at St. Vincent's Hospital. An electrocardiogram (EKG) indicates I am not having a heart attack, but when my blood tests are further analyzed, I am called back to review the results. I have dismissed the episode as anxiety, so when we arrive the next day, my primary concern is to visit the cafeteria and look for donuts. We ride the elevator to the seventh floor to save time.

★　★　★　★　★

When I was in the fifth grade I rode the same elevator almost every day, my destination the second-floor hospital cafeteria. There, they had the longest strips of bacon I had ever seen, eggs fried with crispy edges, French toast with cinnamon, and fruit juice in flavors I had never tasted before (we only had apple juice at home, in brown glass gallon-jugs from the orchard across the street). The best treats were the glazed donuts. Each bite was sweet and gooey; the brushed sugar coating and warm dough melting in my mouth. I always took two.

A free, all-you-could-eat breakfast was the reward for serving the six o'clock morning mass. I usually walked the nine blocks to the hospital chapel, carrying a flashlight to cut the dark stretches of the neighborhood. I had to arrive by 5:45 a.m. to help the grumpy priest into his garments: he would be upset if I was a minute late. After mass, and after drinking my last cup of hot chocolate, I had time to linger while walking the half-mile to St. Mary of the Angels, the nearby Catholic school.

In spring, before school was over, I rode my bike to the hospital. The faithful calls of mourning doves, sitting as pairs along the power lines, always shared my route. In the fall, when the chill mornings held the smell of burning leaves, I stopped to throw horse chestnuts down the streets, sometimes aiming at Halloween pumpkins on doorsteps. Vince Lombardi was the coach of the Packers, Bart Starr was throwing touchdown passes, and football-festive green and gold decorations lined the neighborhoods until late November.

In early winter, when heavy curtains of wet snow drifted through the streetlights, I pretended I was inside a snow globe. When it turned bitterly cold—smoke from the chimneys going straight up into the night, tight snow squeaking beneath my boots—my mom would try to give me a ride. But if my dad was working the midnight shift at the power plant and had our family's only car, I simply bundled up, leaning sideways against the cutting wind that bit my cheeks and numbed my face. I never wore the scarves my grandma knit; I hated how the cloth always got wet from my breath and pieces of wool stuck to my tongue.

My mom told her bridge club friends that I never complained about nasty weather or getting up so early in the morning when my friends were still asleep. I was unknowingly gaining good traits for the wildlife biologist I would become.

★ ★ ★ ★ ★

Today, the elevator doors open into a waiting area that has the decor and soft furniture of a hotel lobby. It exudes a warmth uncharacteristic of what I would expect in any hospital. The few elderly patients are being served coffee, and cookies are handy on a side table. The sign overhead says Department of Oncology.

Are we in the right place?

As a wildlife biologist, I know many similar "-ology" words: ornithology (birds), mammalogy, herpetology (snakes and reptiles), ichthyology (fish), parasitology. Likewise, medical terms like physiology, neurology, and hematology were commonly used in many of my university courses. Perhaps oncology is a unique term used in hospitals to describe the study of tropical medicine.

Dr. Saphner's nurse waves to us. She apologizes; the doctor will be a few minutes late. She assures us he will be with us shortly, as if waiting for him is somehow an offense.

"Can I do anything to make you more comfortable? A coffee or juice?"

"Hmm, we're fine."

Aren't we?

Soon we are chatting with Dr. Saphner in another plush room. He asks about our visit to the city and our recent stay in Costa Rica without any indication he needs to limit his time with us.

He slips easily into questions about my parents and siblings, particularly what I know about their medical histories. I assume documenting family history is standard procedure for new patients. Our history is unremarkable. We are all healthy.

Then Dr. Saphner casually states that my blood test has revealed some abnormalities.

"Your white blood cell count is over 17,000. While a simple blood test alone is not conclusive evidence, it is highly indicative of chronic lymphocytic leukemia, or CLL. Prolymphocytic leukemia, or PLL, is also a possibility, but there are too many cell fragments in the sample for a proper diagnosis."

"What is the normal level for white blood cells?" I ask, too confused by the terms he has used to ask anything else.

"A range of 4,000 to 10,000 would be considered normal," he says.

"Maybe the high white blood cell count means I have mononucleosis. I have been quite tired for several weeks," I reply.

"Not in this case, Mr. Herzog. Your count is too high and I suspect the abnormal lymphocytes are continuing to increase. If you did have mononucleosis, your white blood cell count would be declining by now."

"What if I had a different type of infection, could my white blood cells also increase?"

"Certainly," replies Dr. Saphner.

"What about a tropical disease or infection?"

"I imagine WBC counts could rise, but you would have to consult a specialist in tropical medicine. Unfortunately, we have no one with that expertise here in Green Bay."

He wishes us well and strongly advises us to pursue further testing as soon as we return to Alberta. A copy of his preliminary report will be waiting for us tomorrow.

My wife and I talk about the uncertainty of the results as we approach the elevator. CLL? PLL? Neither of us relates these acronyms to leukemia or even remotely to a diagnosis of cancer. What the hell does "lymphocytic" mean, anyway? As we try to unravel the news, we forget to stop at the cafeteria.

My youngest sister, Kathy, works in the accounting office at the hospital. Maybe she knows about oncology and why we were at that odd department.

I ask her that night at dinner. She takes me aside and tells me, "The department of oncology is for cancer care."

Cancer? Saphner hadn't said anything about cancer. He never said *that* word. My health had been excellent in Costa Rica, better than that of my local friends. Not even a case of diarrhea or a bout of stomach flu caught me, despite my fondness for the food and *refrescos* (fresh fruit smoothies prepared with tap water) at roadside cantinas. Not even a sore throat or headache. Only the mysterious fatigue.

I am at the pinnacle of my career and eager to return to Costa Rica. I am not sick. I don't get sick. I have *never* been sick.

Cancer? What kind of *bullshit* is this?

My wife and I tell our families the blood tests are inconclusive and that I am only adjusting to the effects of travel, stress, and the shock of winter. I promise to see my family doctor as soon as we return home. Now is not the time to worry. Now is the time to celebrate Christmas.

Chapter 3
Denial

These guys should be a little more sensitive to the fact that not everyone who comes in here has cancer. Obviously there has been some kind of a mix-up.

–Alan Hobson, *Climb Back from Cancer*

A few days after we arrive home, I meet our family doctor, Dr. Mason (he is treating my daughter for a case of dehydration). He is pleased to hear of my good health in Costa Rica, but says I need to see him for a routine physical exam, emphasizing that it is important for his records. I don't want to see him until I can unravel the unsettling information from Wisconsin, but he insists that he has time to see me next week. I relent, but leave the copy of my results in the back pocket of my jeans when I undress for my examination.

Dr. Mason finds nothing overtly unhealthy about me. Only when he orders a standard blood test do I reluctantly give him the report, and then only as he is walking down the hallway to his next appointment. I tell him I am handing it over strictly as a professional courtesy to the doctor in Green Bay (who has written that I am a nice person with an interesting disease).

Perhaps the findings from Wisconsin are related to my change of diet since leaving Costa Rica. I am no longer eating vitamin-laden fruits like mango, papaya, and guava every day. Apples, oranges, and winter vegetables (the hunter food of my youth) must be woefully poor substitutes for maintaining my immune system, therefore, I eat an abundance of coconuts and plantains, and gorge on pineapple several days before complying with the new blood test.

The result? My white cell count (WBC) has risen to 21,000 and again reveals atypically large and malformed white blood cells. The analysis further suggests I have CLL, a cancer of the bone marrow, the spongy tissue that fills the centers of my bones.

Dr. Mason is unhappy with my attempt at secrecy and doesn't hesitate to use the word "cancer." I resist his diagnosis, saying I must have a tropical disease or infection—even parasites—that are unknown in Canada. I suggest a doctor with experience in tropical medicine will dispel any notions of cancer.

Instead, he refers me to a Dr. Snyder in Calgary. His specialty is also oncology. Surely, I am being misdirected again.

★ ★ ★ ★ ★

Dr. Snyder also wants to stick me with cancer.

"I suspect you have CLL, or chronic lymphocytic leukemia, a cancer of the blood and bone marrow," he says, looking down at the papers on his desk. "Typically it is a cancer found in older people, sixty-five to seventy years of age. Cases are rare in individuals less than forty years old."

"I am only forty-one," I say, lifting my shoulders and spreading my hands in disbelief.

"Well," he counters without making eye contact, "no one is immune from cancer."

"Maybe I caught malaria or yellow fever while I was in Costa Rica."

"Those diseases are obviously out of the question in your case," he answers.

"I was also in Belize, Honduras and Guatemala—how about dengue fever or the kissing bug disease? Charles Darwin caught that."

No comment. He glances at me briefly while flipping the pages in his file.

I am sitting across from him in a chair that sits low to the floor. I feel small and vulnerable.

"I recently handled tranquilized monkeys in the jungle," I say, hoping to spark his interest in something besides a diagnosis of cancer.

More sorting of papers.

"I had a bad case of chiggers, skin parasites, and recently a biologist I was working with got peppered with nematodes after handling jaguar scats. I don't think I touched them, but I did share meals with park guards who had something called cat scratch fever. What do you know about those possibilities?"

My voice is rising. I know I could *kick his ass* on any trail of his choosing.

I am about to add that there was a cholera epidemic in Costa Rica when, sighing heavily, Dr. Snyder leans back into his chair, crosses his arms, and finally stares directly at me.

"You have cancer, Mr. Herzog, and looking for other explanations is only a type of denial. You might even have prolymphocytic leukemia (PLL), which is a more aggressive kind. My diagnosis will be evident *if* you go for a bone marrow biopsy tomorrow."

He jabs a form at me across the desk, head down as if I do not exist. I snatch the paper rudely from his hand. I will get the biopsy just so he can see that some obscure tropical health problem is mimicking what he thinks is cancer. Monkey saliva, jungle fever, bites from army ants . . . it just has to be something else.

★ ★ ★ ★ ★

Months pass as I wait for the biopsy results. I try to concentrate on the daily events of our lives—my daughters are in new schools, my wife has restarted her studies, and I am at work, discussing my tropical wildlife studies and learning of new developments at the college—but I can't shake the notion that has persisted since those days in the Northwoods that I feel less well than I should.

I slowly acknowledge I have none of the typical signs or symptoms I associate with tropical disorders—weight loss, rashes, fevers, or intense bouts of diarrhea—and I finally admit I had been foolish to believe I was simply adjusting to a northern climate.

My biopsy results eventually arrive from Calgary: I do have CLL.

Dr. Mason offers no prediction or forecast of what will happen to me in the future, no mention of possible treatments, no prognosis or odds of survival. No gnashing of teeth, no wringing of hands. He is not offering consolation and I have no tears.

I have cancer. It is just that simple.

A nurse interrupts our meeting to say Dr. Mason is needed at the hospital.

I don't know how to react—I am confused that cancer can be chronic. I thought being told you had cancer meant you only had time to say your good-byes. Apparently, I am not expected to die anytime *soon*.

Chapter 4
Watching Chickens

One must be resigned to waiting: waiting for the
animal to appear, for the rain or snow to stop, for
porters to arrive.

—George Schaller, *A Naturalist and Other Beasts: Tales from*
a Life in the Field

At our next appointment, Dr. Mason emphasizes CLL normally
progresses slowly; some people live with it for years without
complications, often dying of something else. Therefore, the
best course of action is no action at all.

Perhaps I have little to fear. Maybe because I am young and
fit, my CLL will be a slow mover.

But, I tell him, if I have cancer, I *want* action. I want the
problem fixed quickly, like when I broke my arm in the sixth
grade. That was a short stint with a cast my friends admired,
and my grandma bought me a new Hardy Boys book every
week I saw the doctor.

I tell him without treatment, I am no more than a dead
man walking.

Dr. Mason frowns and seems mad at my remark, pulling
hard with both hands on the stethoscope around his neck. I
will just have to learn to accept the disease, he says, and it is
time to move on from my initial attempts at denial, and my

obvious anger about what I consider to be the injustice of not receiving immediate treatment.

"If that's the case," I ask him, "What can I do to inhibit the growth of the disease?"

"There is nothing specific I can recommend. Do what you have always done to maintain good health."

"What about fieldwork?"

He only offers shallow guidance, saying it might be best to avoid infections, injuries and extraordinary activities that might tax my health.

I wonder aloud about when I got leukemia. Was it at some point before moving to Costa Rica? Or was it after the strike of a fer-de-lance bounced off the tough rubber of my boot, or that night a year later when I unknowingly waded chest-deep across a tidal channel full of crocodiles? The park guards got a laugh out of that incident, daring each other (and me) to repeat the feat.

Dr. Mason says no, none of this matters to my future. I am upset he does not offer to look for clues in my file, and I do not find comfort in his matter-of-fact approach to my case, as if I have a virus and I will be healthy again, without treatment, once it has run its course.

He sets my current level of 27,000 WBC as my baseline, and gives me a standing order to report for blood tests every six months to monitor the "progressive accumulation of the functionally incompetent lymphocytes" in my bloodstream. I like the word "incompetent;" it sounds like a reason to believe CLL cannot kill me.

The rule of thumb, he says, is to watch for a doubling of the lymphocyte count between tests, a red flag that will warn us that the rogue white cells are being produced at a danger-ous rate. I also need to report any night sweats, fevers, weight loss, enlarged lymph nodes, pains in my abdomen, or increasing fatigue. I get the notion I should be happy because I do not have any of these problems so far, other than being tired.

I have my walking papers and I'm told to *watch and wait*, the only advice given to patients diagnosed with CLL.

I feel I need to hunker down despite clear skies, a massive storm somewhere over the horizon that will strike before I see its leading edge. So, a few days later, I decide to accept a recent offer from the college to become the chairperson of my department. The position is a demanding office job, but by keeping me close to home, it will reduce the wear and tear of fieldwork until I can see how my body reacts to the cancer within me.

Watch and wait. I *know* when it is worthwhile to watch and wait—when you wait to witness spectacular moments of insight into an animal's life, and build vibrant memories of nature's secrets. When you lift your head to search the night sky for the Southern Cross, waiting for the tide to rise so you can watch sea turtles crawl onto their nesting beaches. Or when you patiently watch a grizzly sow and her cubs playfully dig up tundra plants, the wind tickling their dark, shiny hair as you wait to ascend the mountain safely. Or when you wait for prairie chickens to cackle in the dark.

★ ★ ★ ★ ★

I was at the wildlife department at 4:00 a.m. There were seven of us, and we were driven out of town under a moonless sky, weaving along sandy back roads, with nothing but flat blackness enclosing our headlights. The darkness foretold nothing about the landscape I would be seeing for the first time, and I thought about the chances of screwing up my assignment to count prairie chickens—a species I had never heard of until two days before.

I was left by the side of the road and told to proceed north for a few hundred yards, where I would find an irrigation ditch (being a city boy, I was not sure what to look for). From there I would follow the canal east until it continued to a fence line. There I would turn south, watching for the outline of a small canvas blind in the middle of the prairie on my right-hand side.

I had about forty minutes to reach my destination.

It was crucial to be inside my blind before the birds were outside on the booming ground (the name for a traditional spring communal breeding place they used every year). "Booming" is the rhythmic hollow sound created by the males as they expel air from the bright orange skin pouches along their necks. If I arrived late, the birds would scatter and breeding activities would stop, perhaps for several days. The species only survived in Wisconsin in a few isolated areas and was listed as an endangered species. Disturbing them could be costly to their breeding success.

Getting lost—a possibility voiced by the other novice observers—did not concern me; my dad had taught me to use a compass. I was only worried about walking too slowly or missing a landmark.

I set my bearing, pointing the beam of my flashlight to the north. I walked briskly, wearing canvas pants and a stout winter coat over nylon fleece, top and bottom. The canal proved easy to find because the willow saplings along its border whipped me in the face several times in the dark. Twenty-five minutes to go.

I was dressed for ice-fishing, not hiking. I started to worry that I would freeze when I sat in the blind, so in a futile effort to stop sweating, I started blowing air down the inside of my shirt as I walked. I finally decided to shed my insulated underwear, which involved standing barefoot on the frozen ground, nearly naked, while I redressed. Ten minutes left on the clock.

The fence crossing the canal was soon visible in the tiny band of yellow light sneaking up the horizon. As I hiked south, I repeatedly crouched low to the ground as I had been told, looking for a square silhouette rising above the darkness still sticking to the field.

Where was it? How much farther? Only ten minutes to go. Was I in the right place? That dark shape—that must be it.

I tripped on a mound of dirt as I ran across the field, my spare clothes scattering ahead of me. I scrambled inside the blind, eventually finding my notebook, binoculars and camera, thankful it was still quiet outside.

Then the sound of wingbeats landing on the ground. Hooting sounds to the right. Quiet again. Then the rustling of feathers, much closer. Then the pounding of feet, and then, deep booming sounds resonate throughout the blind.

I peeked through a tiny slit in the canvas to begin counting the birds; the nearest male, barely feet away, had stopped displaying in the sparkling grass and was staring at me. He stomped a few feet away to challenge his rivals, but I was certain he kept his eye on me throughout the frosty morning.

I skipped classes to spend another six mornings in the field that spring. And during the next two years, I would be the one driving volunteers to observe the birds in the predawn hours, racing to the campus later in the mornings, trying to stay awake in warm classrooms while clad in long johns. By then I had met the Hamerstroms, the famous prairie chicken biologists who had been trained by the legendary conservationist Aldo Leopold. I was twenty-one years old, eager to watch and wait.

★   ★   ★   ★   ★

I look up the definition of "cope," the word most often used by doctors while counseling their patients. I had always thought it meant muddling through, but I learn that the definition is more like "being able to deal successfully with a problem or a sustained crisis." I am Dr. Mason's only patient with CLL and I suspect he has little experience with the disease. There is no cancer department at the local hospital, and the only support group is restricted to breast cancer survivors. I will not be able to see the local oncologist until I truly get sick. I feel alone, without a clear line of sight into the uncertainties of my condition.

If I am to cope, I need to learn how bone marrow functions, what causes CLL to erupt, how it progresses, and the scope of current treatments and their success.

I once taught courses in human biology to nursing students. I dig out my notes on cell biology and read that bone marrow contains hematopoietic, or blood-forming, stem cells that make white blood cells, red blood cells and platelets. These cells can only make blood and are not the same as embryonic stem cells, which develop into every type of cell in the body.

On-line I read that CLL occurs when there is genetic damage to blood-stem cells which causes the uncontrolled production of enlarged and misshaped white blood cells or lymphocytes. These leukemic or "cancer" cells do not mature normally and fail to die when they should, allowing them to build up in huge numbers in the bone marrow. They crowd out healthy white and red blood cells, and reduce the number of blood-clotting platelets. Eventually they leave the marrow (as do normal blood cells), invading the circulatory system; this is the cause of my high WBC counts.

The abnormal white blood cells do not fight infection, and the bastards often impair the function of other organs in the body. By reducing the number of red blood cells and platelets, they can cause easy bleeding. CLL offers me a cheerless trifecta: rampant infection, organ failure, and even bleeding to death, in no particular fashion, before I reach the end of the trail.

What about treatment? I'm still angry Dr. Mason had nothing to offer, nothing to share about how I might be treated in the future.

I should be able to find out what is being done to treat CLL: I routinely read scientific articles and technical wildlife studies, and I know how to obtain the details of studies written by specialists buried in obscure publications and old files in libraries. Cancer studies must be written using comparable terms and analysis and be available in similar places.

I only find a few reports. I learn that early intervention to treat patients in good health typically aggravates rather than stops CLL (hence the concept of watch and wait). Likewise, chemotherapy has not proven effective in inducing remission, and people often die from the complications created by such treatment.

I do not find any overlooked cures for the disease (I didn't expect to uncover one), but I am disappointed there are no recommendations to use vitamins, herbs or special foods or diets to slow the progress of the disease. Fortunately, new chemotherapy protocols are being investigated at hospitals in the United States and Europe.

I do discover that because my only evidence of CLL is a high level of lymphocytes, I am at the lowest level (Stage 0) in the Rai system that rates the severity of CLL. The system ends at Stage 4, when I would be considered high-risk with too few blood platelets, enlarged lymph nodes, spleen, or liver, and the likelihood of anemia. I assume the intermediate levels will be opportunities for treatment long before the dangers of Stage 4.

Within a month of meeting with Dr. Mason, I've gathered a large three-ring binder filled with information, put sticky tabs on the pages to update while watching and waiting, and highlighted my questions in yellow for my next appointment in six months' time. For the time being, I have smothered my worries and anger with facts.

Chapter 5

Down the River

Spending time in nature, particularly wilderness, can pose physical dangers, but rejecting nature because of those risks and discomforts is a greater gamble.

—Richard Louv, *The Nature Principle*

Knowledge about my cancer helps defuse the lethal power of the word. I now have a strategy: I will learn to interpret the results of my ongoing blood tests, I will monitor my physical condition for the signs and symptoms of CLL, and I will continue my research into the disease.

It is a rational plan and I hope time is on my side, but if I were embarking on a rafting trip (instead of a journey with cancer), I feel I would still be heading downriver into trouble without a decent map. Now the water is quiet, the wind calm. But rapids, rocks, whirlpools, sweepers, and waterfalls lie somewhere ahead.

The unpredictable and nebulous nature of CLL makes it hard to explain my condition to my parents and siblings in Wisconsin. I repeatedly dismiss any notions that I might die, insisting my age and health ensure few complications in the future. And if I need treatment, I assure them, medical science will come to the rescue.

I do not tell my colleagues I have cancer, wanting to maintain my stature among them, and I only casually tell my best friends, not wanting them to worry about me, wanting them to see me as they always have. I choose to be secretive; I do not want to be known as being tagged by cancer.

As for my young daughters (only four and six years old), my wife and I decide they are too young to understand how I could be sick when I look so well, and I want to shield them from ever having to worry about me. I will disguise my concerns as I long as I can to ensure their lives are carefree and happy.

How does my wife react? My illness adds more stress to a gap in our marriage. She left her home, family, job, and comfortable surroundings in Green Bay to share her life with me. The transition has remained difficult over the years, and I feel responsible for her happiness. Despite my diagnosis, I feel I am still the primary caregiver in our relationship.

I push ahead alone, concentrating on making our lives happy and worry-free, planning time outdoors for hiking, skiing and camping. For now, the many soft days afield replace the rugged weeks I formerly spent doing fieldwork in the bush. I do not miss them yet because it is a precious time: I lose myself in nature, seeing its wonders as I did as a boy through the eyes of my girls.

I receive an invitation to return to Costa Rica to study the macaws. It hurts to decline. I will miss the excitement and satisfaction of working in the tropics, but because my immune system is impaired, even simple scratches and bug bites from the jungle might lead to costly infections. It seems unfair, especially because I've been stable since returning home.

★　★　★　★　★

I remain in Stage 0 for the next three years, continuing to have a "good" cancer. If I wake up hot in bed, it is simply too many blankets, not night sweats. If I feel chilled indoors on a winter day, I wear a sweater to dispel my thoughts of cancer-induced fevers. I watch my weight—I stay within a few pounds downside of 155. Only in hindsight, do I notice that I am fooled by bursts of energy that hide the steady decline in my stamina, and that I have become an easy target for lengthy (and harsh) colds and flus for the first time in my life.

The dots I put on my chart of bi-annual blood tests hover between 30,000 and 38,000 WBC. I adopt a "see no evil, hear no evil" mentality and threaten to stop filling my standing order. Dr. Mason reminds me I am already being cocky by skipping my tests, sometimes by several weeks (I tease the technicians, asking them to submit my results from the previous months with new dates, but they reluctantly refuse my tempting offers of free pizza and beer).

Perhaps he suspects that when I miss my tests, I gain the illusion of control over my disease by deciding when it can make itself evident. If so, he is correct. And after the tests are done, I try to postpone our appointments because they cast dark shadows across my days.

I often feel like life is going on without me. I would much rather be watching and waiting for wonderful things, like coyote pups finally emerging from their den after I've waited nearby, hiding silently for hours, in wet, mosquito-infested grass. Even waiting for rescue years ago on the coast of Belize after a massive tropical storm, running out of beans, rice, and beer, in that order, seems preferable to waiting for the shock of a blood test that indicates cancer is on a rampage throughout my body. I hope that day never comes, or is so far in the future that medical science will have a cure for CLL (there has been no encouragement yet from my research).

At times, I can dismiss CLL as a danger lurking inside me. After all, *terciopelos* did not hide along every trail in the jungle.

But then CLL escapes from the wraps of my immune system: my WBC count spikes to 68,000. Only a measly 2,000 short of a fateful double in six months.

Maybe my rising count has been caused by a recent one-two punch: a deep sinus cold and concurrent ear infection of near-infinite duration (I don't recall ever having such a potent combination). I check my research for a correlation between CLL and rampant nose and ear infections, but find none—Dr. Mason says a virus has been hitting his patients.

He shortens the interval of my standing order to three months.

I feel no different, but CLL is spreading. How much time do I have before I am too sick to spend days in the field?

I think of Aldo Leopold and his words in the *Sand County Almanac:* "There are some who can live without wild things and some who cannot. I am one who cannot."

Maybe the upcoming spring will be my last chance to work with wild things. I begin to search for a field project close to home.

Chapter 6

Rapids

Down the river again, a river becoming colder, wider, siltier all the time. A broad stream with braided channels, some navigable and some not; it keeps the boatmen alert.

−Edward Abbey, *Notes from a Cold River*

When I discover a two-year study to census a variety of songbirds (warblers, tanagers, thrushes, sparrows, chickadees, and meadowlarks) near the Old Man River west of Fort Macleod, I am overjoyed at my good fortune, although I know the fieldwork will be tough.

Survey plots are scattered across many square miles of steep, roadless country. Most of the plots are a quarter mile apart, interrupted by rugged terrain. To reach the plots by dawn when the birds start singing, I will need to rise at 3:00 a.m. The pace of work each day will also have to be brisk; surveys must be finished by mid-morning.

The peak breeding season is a run of only six weeks in May and June. And because songbirds are not reliably active in inclement weather, I will need ideal days in the field: no fog, no rain, and few chinooks—fierce winds that barrel down the mountains. High winds mean I will not be able to detect the birds singing at the outer edges of my plots (I listen for ten minutes at each site before racing to the next one, where I listen again), and could derail my best efforts, often for days.

Even with good weather, it is a tight schedule. I will need to bust my ass.

Despite the excitement of going back to the field, I decide it will be prudent to conserve my energy. I promise myself I will go slowly, be wary of overexertion, pace myself: I convince myself I will take naps after fieldwork instead of going fishing or exploring the nearby mountains. I pack one of my three favorite books, *Desert Solitaire* by Edward Abbey, to help me recapture the spirit of the wilderness without leaving camp. If I do get restless, I won't have far to walk to watch prairie falcons hunt gophers, or collect the specimens I need to refresh my knowledge of the local flora.

I charge ahead the first few mornings, pinching myself while brewing my coffee when the stars are still brilliant, untouched by the hint of dawn. After the years of office work, the lung-busting hiking is a struggle, and I am breathless and behind schedule each morning. I revise the design of the study to be less strenuous, but even with perfect weather, I cannot complete the surveys alone on time. I hire a former student to do the last two rounds of counts at the most difficult sites, and fortunately, the mountains hold the storms at high elevation. I am winded and bruised by the end of the field season, but renewed in spirit and pleased with the high quality of our data.

Being in the wild allows me to forget about cancer. When I hurry between plots, I scan the sky for changes in the weather, almost heedless of where I put my feet. When I listen for birds, only the slight variations in their songs fill my mind.

Later in the day, I watch ravens sweep along the cliffs above the river, and the grizzly that digs plants near camp. I go to bed once I hear the coyotes bark and yip under the traveling moon, and wake unburdened by the effort to be normal at the college and home.

My immune system holds up to the rigors of fieldwork, so I stop worrying about the ticks that carry Rocky Mountain spotted fever. And when my family joins me as I collate data, we have a tremendous week of camping, roasting marshmallows by the fire, picking wild berries, and smashing rocks along the river looking for geodes.

I am feeling well for the first time since being blindsided by cancer. When my blood test in early July shows a drop of 2,000 to 66,000 WBC, I rejoice. I've always felt that fieldwork and the power of nature are potent forces strengthening my body and mind, and now I have proof, even though the decrease is numerically insignificant (a fact I easily ignore).

Perhaps it is time to rethink the decisions I have made over the past few years to avoid the physical challenges of field studies. Maybe when I finish the bird study I will go back in the field full-time. Maybe even find out how the macaws are doing.

Hope reigns.

★　★　★　★　★

October. Three months later. A WBC count of 82,000. Dammit, how did this happen? I'm still feeling good; there has been no change that I can see or feel.

I walk to the edge of the coulees and stare at Chief Mountain in the distance. I had been hopefully confident that the strength I had acquired from counting songbirds would protect me from any further increases in my counts. I had allowed myself to imagine stable numbers would return for months and years, and that I would have a new future filled with fieldwork and adventure. I am angry at having deceived myself.

The interval between my blood tests is reduced to two months. I begin to search my body for lumps.

★ ★ ★ ★ ★

December. A count of 112,000 WBC. The CLL is spreading through my body like an invasive species. Usually harmless in their native environment, invasive species settle in new locales and, following a lull after the initial period of settlement, often cause widespread damage to existing flora and fauna. The consequences thereafter are often catastrophic. Examples abound: Burmese pythons and now Nile crocodiles in Florida, Asian carp in the Mississippi River, zebra and quagga mussels in the Great Lakes, rats and pigs driving birds to extinction in Hawaii, ever-present Dutch elm disease, purple loosestrife, Scotch broom, killer bees, fire ants . . .

At least now I can legitimately see the local oncologist. Certainly, he will explain why CLL is on the move and what we need to do now.

★ ★ ★ ★ ★

I am told the doctor's workload is immense and my initial appointment is postponed for two weeks. My case must be a low priority; at my next appointment, I wait for two hours until the office closes for the day. When I finally meet the specialist in the new year, I am told there is no reason to start treatment because I have not progressed past Stage 0. He stands and tells me to continue seeing Dr. Mason, rushing out the door before I can open my binder of notes. But for me, "watch and wait", or the new phrase "watchful waiting", is over. Waiting has been replaced by worrying.

Two months later, my blood sample is loaded with 154,000 white blood cells, a strong double in only four months. I have exceeded the benchmark for proliferation.

I plead with Dr. Mason to find me a different oncologist, one who can spend time with me, one willing to discuss the knowledge I have gained about CLL and the new options for treatment. Finally, I head north to meet the experts at the Tom Baker Cancer Centre in Calgary, Alberta, a facility I did not know existed.

Three doctors are waiting when I arrive and, after we shake hands, they impress me immediately by asking what is in my binder. Inside I have every medical article, report, and publication I have acquired in the past five years. The first page is the chart I have made of all my WBC counts since diagnosis. I have copies which I pass around the table. Dr. Russell smiles, saying they have never had a prospective patient with such a detailed case history of his own cancer.

"It is extremely difficult to predict the progress of CLL," he says, "but I see you know that from your notes. You are also correct that early intervention often accelerates the course of the disease. We don't know why at this time."

I ask about the nature of my escalating counts. "Certainly the recent increase in your counts is unsettling, but I do not find them significantly ominous to push for immediate treatment," he replies, adding that it was fortunate I had avoided the complications experienced by many patients with CLL by remaining at Stage 0 for so long. My counts, however, *will rise*, rate unknown.

When I ask for an absolute number on which to base the need for treatment, Dr. Russell says that there is no finite level for how high counts can go before they dictate intervention. Somehow, perhaps from the tone of his answer, I suspect 200,000, maybe 250,000 might do it, even if I remain at Stage 0.

I mention the poor success of treating CLL with conventional chemotherapy in the studies I have in my binder. I ask about new research underway at hospitals in Europe and the United States, particularly the use of monoclonal antibodies that only kill cancer cells. While the doctors agree that this is a very exciting approach, it will take years of additional research to refine suitable treatments.

"Why don't we have your siblings tested for compatibility as potential bone marrow donors?" asks one of the doctors. "You might be a good candidate because of your age and good health."

The information I have on bone marrow transplants describes low rates of success, but I am told that my data are unreliable and outdated by several years. New techniques are available and in use at the centre, with promising results. Our conversation extends beyond an hour and I find myself listening to the comments they share between them as if I am a colleague.

I now have expert doctors willing to monitor my file, and they will receive copies of all tests ordered by either my local oncologist or family doctor. I have two brothers and three sisters who may be able to donate bone marrow (I later learn the chances of a sibling match are one in four).

As the meeting ends, the doctors encourage me to continue my bird studies. One of them asks me how I study birds, wondering how I can collect information on such elusive creatures. I am surprised by his interest, and happier still to know he is on my team.

I am no longer alone as CLL gains ground on me. And I find out a few months later that Kathy, the youngest member of our family (born eleven years after me), is a bone marrow match. I do not know what that means, but I am happy to know she is there.

* * * * *

I start the second year of the bird study a few months later, confident my familiarity with the study area (and the moral support of my doctors) will help ensure a successful field season. I tire, however, within days, and despite big naps, protein drinks, and extra vitamins, I am barely able to do half of the surveys required each day. I am behind schedule, worried the high WBC count I carry with me (now at 196,000—42,000 more than when I met the doctors in Calgary) is the cause of my decline.

With the study in danger, I search for help. Three songbird biologists working in the area make time to join me. Although the weather is good, and we collect all the data, I do not have a single day of fun in the field.

While breaking camp, I believe that my days afield in the wild are likely over. CLL, a nefarious SOB, has struck me down and will *always* find new ways to track me, even in the shelter of nature. By late summer my WBC count has ripped ahead to 258,000. When I visualize what the leukemia must be doing to my body, I see the weepy, jelly-like marrow I have seen in the long bones of deer and antelope that have starved to death in the grip of winter.

I casually report the news to our families in Wisconsin. Their concern is genuine, but only a month ago many of them saw me whooping it up during a three-week visit at the Herzog cabin. And now my mom also has cancer.

My oncologist in Lethbridge wants to put me on chlorambucil. It is an old medication: several studies I have read confirm it has poor long-lasting results. The drug also destroys healthy human cells; especially those of the skin and other organs, and many oncologists believe it can cause CLL to become drug-resistant and induce surviving cells to become more aggressive.

If true, I suspect that chemotherapy with chlorambucil might impact my chances of a bone marrow transplant.

I counter his recommendation with the innovative cutting-edge options for treatment available in Calgary, and the upcoming results of clinical trials elsewhere that I have discovered in my research. When he forces a grin, I insist we must use the newer drugs I *know* are being used with good success.

Any confidence I might have had in his ability to help me vanishes when he concedes a sense of helplessness, telling me that had he known beforehand how many of his patients were destined to die, he would not have switched his career from welding to medicine.

I refuse the treatment. Besides, its toxic ingredients are a blend of mustard derivatives. My grandpa inhaled mustard gas in World War I, and lived with chronic lung problems before dying of liver cancer at a young age. I do not want that crap in my body.

I call the Tom Baker Cancer Centre for help and soon become very angry.

Chlorambucil is my only option because Alberta Health Services insists on its use as the first line of treatment for CLL. Bureaucrats are dictating my treatment instead of the foremost cancer doctors in the province, who are known internationally for their work. I want to push back but do not know how, so when the snow comes, I start the drug, trying not to think of poison when swallowing the ugly yellow pills four times a day.

★ ★ ★ ★ ★

January. The seventh year since my diagnosis. I can no longer maintain my regular pace of life. There are no longer any normal days.

I feel unsteady and at times nauseated with the chlorambucil destroying cells throughout my body, but the chemotherapy rapidly lowers my counts. When my test in April indicates a count of only 19,000 WBC after six months, I fulfill the government's mandate of a reduction to 25,000. I quit taking the drug, but I am not hopeful my positive response will deliver long-term success—too much research states otherwise, and the best protocols are heading in other directions.

My uneasiness is not unfounded; my counts double to 49,000 in three months. Chlorambucil is the bust I feared it would be at the outset and I am furious that it will likely unleash an even more virulent resurgence of CLL. My mind is overwhelmed with "what-if" scenarios, overloaded with anxiety about the future. I feel the end of my life coming toward me, one step at a time.

I cancel a river trip I had been planning all winter, and when I return in the fall to full-time work at the college, I lack the energy to walk the three flights of stairs to my office (despite the switchbacks I employ). I tire readily by mid-morning, and try to compensate for my reduced effectiveness on the job by staying after hours and returning to work on weekends, believing that if I only had one more hour or one more day, I could complete my never-ending list of duties.

There is no time for nature.

Every morning my wife finds me propped up on one elbow as I struggle to get out of bed on time for work. There are no Friday nights on the town: I am too weak and always tense. I pull back from acting spontaneously, making decisions only after diligently comparing choices, only to try and reverse them later. Trying to squeeze life from every day, I am unable to follow my gut feelings.

As my health declines, I feel even more responsible for the happiness of my family, frantically struggling to make every moment perfect for them. Because I have almost no tolerance for disagreements and stress, I am also trying, unknowingly, to control the emotions of everyone in the family, wanting to have total peace as a refuge from the rising uncertainty.

Things are going wrong. I want to lie to my doctors, say I am drenched with night sweats, my weight dropping like a stone. I almost hope to find lumps bulging under my armpits. How else will I get the best treatment before it is too late, and escape from the long ordeal of watching and waiting that now threatens to become toxic with depression?

Chapter 7

Whirlpools

On a big, steep river, the water thundered into a hole with such force that, should you inadvertently tip your craft into one, it could pull you, your life jacket, and your kayak down . . . endlessly recirculating you as the water spins through the hole. This is known as a "keeper."

–Peter Stark, *Last Breath: The Limits of Adventure*

When I awake, roll to the side of the mattress, and swing my legs over the side of the bed, the skin on the right side of my groin feels taut, and there is something solid underneath the surface. A bulge the size of a small lemon has appeared overnight, pushing from the inside out, the hard mass refusing to move when I try to shift its position. Maybe I have a hernia, but there is no pain.

The lump appears two weeks before Christmas. A week later I lie on a biopsy table, seven years and a day since that fateful visit to the doctor at St. Vincent's. My results will be ready at the start of the new year.

A few days later, the incision in my groin still hurts, but I want to enjoy our family's favorite holiday tradition of zipping down the local ski hill on sleds and saucers. These outings are followed by mugs of hot chocolate with whipped cream on top—the silly stuff that comes in a spray can that you can squirt into your mouth (and get on your face). Surely, I can avoid falling and tearing the stitches in my leg when I walk up the Sugar Bowl, the local hill. When I am finally convinced that sledding is a foolish idea, we go to the indoor water park.

I want the girls to have fun, and I know they will be worried if I only sit poolside on the lounge chairs, so I slowly climb the stairs to the highest tube, placing both feet on each step. I sit with my hands in my lap as I ride down to the pool, adding pressure to the wad of bandages over my incision (no one thinks about bacteria in the water infecting my wound, least of all me). But after a few runs, I decide to stop and watch my daughters ride, swim, and splash each other. I struggle to enjoy the contests they are having holding their breath underwater: they are so young and happy. I feel myself hoping that the lump is benign, or something else unrelated to cancer.

After hot chocolate, I reread the articles in my binder that imply that if the hard mass is an enlarged lymph node or tumor, I have advanced to Stage 1. I do not have the night sweats, fevers or weight loss I believe are associated with Stage 2. I have no pain, and because this is my first obvious physical sign of having CLL, I continue to assume Stages 2 to 4 will be on my horizon, hopefully a distant one.

What will Dr. Mason say tomorrow? Will he have notified my doctors in Calgary?

Late the next day, the surgeon who performed the biopsy enters the waiting room, obviously uneasy and nervous to be seeing me. Why is he here? Where in the hell is Dr. Mason? What else could he be doing at this critical moment?

"Is there someone with you?" asks Dr. Grant, surprised I am alone.

"No," I reply, putting down the newest issue of the wildlife magazine I have brought from home. "I'm good meeting you on my own."

"I have your results," he says, opening his folder. "They indicate you have diffuse large B-cell lymphoma, or Richter's transformation. B-cell lymphoma is a severe condition, indeed life-threatening. I'm very sorry to be giving you such difficult news, especially during the holidays," he says, glancing away from me.

"That's okay." I shrug my shoulders, exhaling with relief. "Let's hope I have the *other* condition, the Richter's thing." It sounds like it has less severe implications, like it will be something more easily tackled.

"When will you be ordering the additional tests?" I ask. "Or will it be Dr. Mason? I'm really busy preparing for the new semester but things will settle down in a couple of weeks," I add, thinking there is no need for urgency.

"Oh, no," he exclaims, quite stricken. "There is no difference in your results; the terms both mean the same thing. You have a very serious cancer. I'm so sorry this has happened to you."

"That is *not* what I heard, Dr. Grant," I say, my voice rising. "You said there are *two* possibilities. I either have the serious lymphoma or something else you called Richter's. There are still two options."

"No," he says, shaking his head, a hand to his forehead. "There are no options; the diagnosis is firm. It is extremely important that you have Dr. Mason phone the Tom Baker Cancer Centre immediately when they open Monday morning." He stands to leave, adding that he will tell the nurse I am welcome to stay in the waiting room a while longer.

I sit quietly, watching the darkness fall outside. If I have lymphoma, do I no longer have CLL? What happened to Stages 2, 3, and 4? I have only had Stage 1 for a week, maybe ten days. Nothing had ever indicated I might leapfrog the stages of CLL.

And I had assumed the waiting, watching, and worrying, was never going to end.

When I leave the clinic, the sidewalk is lit by the yellow glow of the streetlights, the drooping branches of the big elms close above my head. The trees are magnificent specimens, and they remind me of the ones that once shaded the streets I walked to serve mass (now long dead of Dutch elm disease). The wind is picking up; dry leaves swirl along the curb, racing across the street.

I walk a long way beneath the blowing trees, the chinook pounding down the plains. I deliberately miss supper, afraid to arrive home before the girls are in bed.

PART II
OVER THE FALLS

I was never daily or nocturnal, suspended outside the limits of either existence. I was never functionally present nor accountably absent. I lived life out of place.

–Arthur W. Frank,
At the Will of the Body: Reflections on Illness

Chapter 8
At the Brink

One thing that I understood very clearly from her words was that with a transplant, timing was everything. You don't want to wait too long to do the transplant, but you also have to make sure that you time it so that you are ready—mind, body and soul—to take the risk of the procedure.

–Robin Roberts, *Everybody's Got Something*

I have chaired many departmental meetings at the college. Now I find myself sitting again at the head of a large table, this time in a boardroom at the Tom Baker Cancer Centre. I recognize two of the doctors from my last visit. Cups are filled with coffee or tea, but cookies lie quietly uneaten on the plate.

My biopsy has been further analyzed in Calgary. There is no doubt that the lymph node in my groin, and likely others in my lymph system, are malignant, invaded by CLL. I have indeed been derailed by Richter's syndrome, a process that affects only five to ten percent of people with CLL. The change is usually sudden and dramatic.

My doctors assure me that the stress of doing songbird counts has not triggered the transformation. CLL simply does not always follow a linear, step-wise pattern; there can be unexplainable variation in the progress of the disease.

I had grudgingly considered CLL a life sentence, but the hasty research I have done in the past few days seems to indicate Richter's transformation is the death penalty: most patients do not respond well to therapy, and those that do have poor rates of survival (average post-treatment survival is only five to eight months). Traditional bone marrow transplants have usually failed.

I am surprised at how relieved I have become about my dire situation. I finally realize that hiding in a life-as-normal routine has paralyzed my thinking, never allowing me to live life fully. And despite doing research and upgrading my notes, I have never had a plan for treatment—no way to strive for success, no goal to achieve, no chance to escape CLL. I've been stuck at base camp. But now my worsening condition means I will finally have the chance to climb whatever the weather.

How to say it best? I am lofty, surprisingly unburdened, both mentally and physically, the sensation of freedom so peculiar I do not recognize what I feel. I am mildly giddy. I don't know what will happen, but I do know one thing: the time has come to stop living my life with cancer.

But first there is a critical decision to make: there are three options for treatment, each with its unique pros and cons and variable probabilities of success. Before the discussion begins, my wife and I are told quite emphatically that *none* of the choices can be considered a cure: some cancer cells are resistant to all treatment options.

Option 1.
A standard chemotherapy routine called CHOP: a regimen consisting of four drugs—**C**yclophosphamide, **H**ydroxydaunorubicin, **O**ncovin, **P**rednisone. The mix is far more potent (and toxic) than chlorambucil.

The goal will be to kill cancer cells faster than they can reproduce without destroying too many of my healthy cells. Remission after only one round of CHOP is often less than a year, so I will likely receive several treatments, each one delaying my potential to recover. Further downside—CHOP can damage the heart, lungs and nervous system.

We move on quickly.

Option 2.

A donor or allogeneic bone marrow transplant. Kathy would be my donor. She is a perfect genetic match, a "10" because her cells are strongly aligned to mine in each of the ten most important categories.

Despite our exceptional compatibility, I am warned that the procedure is still so new it is considered an *experimental* treatment. And a dangerous one.

One that could kill me.

The high-dose chemotherapy required to purge my cancer-ridden bone marrow will destroy my immune system, making me highly vulnerable to life-threatening infections. I will also be at the risk of fever, bleeding, anemia, damage to vital organs (e.g., heart, kidneys, liver, and lungs) and nutritional deficiencies. And if Kathy's cells fail to settle (a process known as engraftment), or I experience donor rejection, I will die.

It will be an ordeal. But if I survive, this option offers the best potential for a complete remission, even a chance to be cancer-free because I will gain the new cancer-fighting powers of my donor's immune cells.

Option 3.

A self-donor or autologous transplant that avoids the heavy risk of donor rejection. My own stem cells would be collected, cleansed of cancer and returned to my body after I receive chemotherapy. The healthy cells would hopefully settle and restore my immune system. I could also gain a complete remission, although this is far less likely with only a rebuild of my usual immunity. Thus, the possibility of a relapse of my disease is higher than with a donor transplant.

As I compare the possibilities, the room quiet, another option seems possible. Why not try the CHOP drug cocktail first rather than risk either of the transplant procedures? CHOP might sufficiently knock back the Richter's and give me several months, or longer, of partial remission. Thereafter, if my condition worsens, I could do a transplant.

"How about trying the CHOP first?" I ask.

"The difficulty with CHOP is that Richter's lymphoma only responds about half the time," replies Dr. Russell, the chief oncologist. "It basically never controls the disease, and delays treatment with potentially more effective therapy. We therefore risk progressing to the point where you are so sick we can't proceed with the transplant."

"But would a small dose of CHOP improve the success of a transplant?"

"No, there is no evidence at all that giving CHOP prior to transplant for someone like yourself will improve your chances. It is simply extra chemotherapy that you would have to endure. We certainly could give you one cycle of CHOP now, if that would make you feel more comfortable, but no more than that."

While I ponder his response, Dr. Russell adds "As you decide, be sure to consider the risks you are taking. There will be no turning back."

I sense the self-donor transplant sacrifices success for safety. CHOP is a long shot.

The usual cut-off age for a donor transplant is fifty. I am forty-eight years old. My body is being damaged daily by Richter's. Time is not on my side.

If I am to succeed, I must stop relying on hope—hope my blood counts do not rise, hope fieldwork can make me healthy, hope I will live a long life, hope I will see my daughters grow up. Hope the CHOP will work for me. Forever the optimist.

I did not walk jungle trails *hoping* not to get bitten by snakes. I did not cross icy streams *hoping* to get to the other side. I did not walk alpine meadows *hoping* not to be attacked by grizzly bears. Then I was confident. And I did not give a moment, a moment, to fear.

I had *faith*.

The room is silent; expectations fill the void. The doctors look at me, then at their notes, then at me again (I never do ask them what they would do). I realize I cannot wait to decide, not even a day.

I want to choose life. I want to risk everything to be well again, to be whole again, to be free to love my family without fear.

I don't remember standing, but I'm on my feet, saying: "I want to do the donor transplant."

No one moves from their chairs as they consider what I have said.

Then everyone is in a hurry. Tests are required. Can I stay overnight? Can I be ready to be admitted before the weekend? Can Kathy be in Calgary within a week?

I ask Dr. Russell for my odds of success. He hesitates; the procedure is new, and the data from patients are still preliminary and sketchy for predictions. Knowing the extent of my research, he knows I should understand his reluctance to give me a number.

I do know about the problems of depending on incomplete data. Making guesses without strong evidence is unprofessional, but I still need a number. I assume the odds will be tough to beat, but not as bleak as crossing an avalanche slope to follow cougar tracks to the other side (a risk I always declined).

I wait. Dr. Russell peers at me over the top of the glasses he wears on a string around his neck.

"Maybe 50–50, perhaps slightly less."

We look at each other, separated by only a few feet. I suspect he wonders if I am changing my mind. Does he worry his reply has made me afraid?

"I can *live* with that," I say.

I do not plan on turning back, but walking to the front desk, my knees are weak.

Chapter 9

The Best Patient Ever

Studies give statistical information about prognosis and treatment effectiveness for large groups of people, but there's no way to know in advance how things will turn out for you, and this uncertainty can be maddening.

–Linda E. Carlson and Michael Speca, *Mindfulness-Based Cancer Recovery*

The door of the elevator opens a few steps away from the fray at the front of the main nursing station. White coats (doctors), purple uniforms (nurses), and green smocks (aides) swirl in several directions. A few gaunt patients clad in standard blue-checked hospital-issue robes shuffle past, either towing or pushing IV poles laden with assorted bags of fluid. They seem to be fixed in place as the traffic rushes around them.

Phones ring, charts are passed, and instructions are shouted above the blare of the intercom. Things are happening, and there is an urgency to get them done. I feel a thrum of solid energy and determination, and a tension I would only expect to find in an emergency room. I have yet to move more than a few feet, feeling like an intruder amid so much purpose.

This is Unit 57, my residence in waiting.

A large green chalkboard dominates the nearest wall. It is smudged with the names of patients and their room assignments. I wonder if the rooms with dusty blank spaces mean good or bad news for their former occupants. Beneath the roster are several computers churning out patient data: ultrasounds, x-rays, blood tests, and orders for new medications.

Wheelchairs, gurneys, and stacks of fresh towels and linen line the hallways. Two trolleys are parked nearby and the air holds the queasy smell of pre-heated lunches awaiting distribution. There are no glazed donuts on the menus beside the trays.

Gaining a foothold at the counter, I wait patiently to be noticed by someone as the action swirls around me. I am having a tour of the ward before I am admitted in a few days. There are worn hats and scarves in a tattered cardboard box at my elbow. I wonder why they are there, only realizing at the end of the tour that they are for patients that have lost their hair because of chemotherapy.

My thoughts stray to what I know about wildlife transplants, or more accurately, wildlife translocations, the capture, transport and release of animals from one location to another. They usually fail because animals try to get back home, are killed by predators, or cannot survive in often less-than-ideal habitats. That was the fate of the prairie chickens I released in Wisconsin to establish another population of the dwindling species.

I hope Kathy's cells act more like those of ring-necked pheasants, a species that spread across North America after arriving from China in 1881. Or like those of Canada geese, although the bird is so successful in many areas that unrestrained populations are causing significant environmental damage.

I'm happy Kathy is my donor. Her response to learning of her compatibility was typical of her personality, one that has endeared her to me over the years: "Did I win? I feel like I just won the lottery!"

I have tremendous confidence in the love, humor, and healing power that my little sister is donating to save my life. I am also exceedingly grateful she has forgiven me for making her cry when she was three years old, yelling at her to keep her small legs straight while I jammed on her snow boots at the bottom of the basement stairs. Now, for my sake, she's offering to endure something much more intense.

Besides the potential to restore my immune functions, I know Kathy has instilled in her stem cells an extra tonnage of vitality. Her cells are indeed cancer killers and will seek and destroy the last of the leukemia cells that will try to escape my upcoming chemotherapy.

A nurse eventually finds me at the front desk and we walk by workstations to an exercise area, where I chat with a patient walking on a treadmill. She has high praise for her doctor and the nurses on the ward.

I know my doctors and nurses are among the top-rated transplant teams in North America. I wrote to the best cancer hospitals in Canada and the United States about receiving a bone marrow transplant. Everyone replied that Tom Baker was an elite treatment center. The highest stamp of approval came when I spoke with the chief nurse at the Boston transplant center.

When I told her that I planned to go to Calgary for treatment, she said, "Why would you go anywhere else?" After that, I no longer had doubts that my treatment was going to be anything short of top-shelf, kick-butt, and world-class.

The experts that will be caring for me have a wealth of experience and resources at their disposal, and I am confident extreme measures will be taken at urgent times. And if there is a war to be fought, it will be my doctors who will do the fighting.

I do not like the military jargon proclaiming the war on cancer. The analogy implies that cancer victims must battle to survive, and keep fighting, depleting all their energy no matter the likelihood of success (cancer typically possesses unlimited ammunition and reinforcements). If you win, you are deemed brave and courageous. You have survived the war. The unintended implication is that those who lose have somehow not fought hard enough.

Suddenly I announce, "I am going to be the best patient the unit has ever had. There will be no complaints, no matter what happens to me in the weeks ahead. No fighting, kicking, or screaming. No biting." And I think to myself, no quiet whimpering.

My guide says nothing about my claim, most likely aware that I have no idea what is going to happen to me. But I am still overcome by that sublime sense of relief that swept over me when I left the boardroom. After pushing hard with my body and soul for seven years, I might as well be awakening on a perfect day to ascend Mount Everest. I have a sole purpose in life: to get well. And I will get there.

The adjacent hallway leads to a small kitchen with a refrigerator filled with juices and ice cream, a sitting room for privacy, rooms for patients, and a large common area overlooking the Bow River. There is a fine panoramic view of downtown Calgary extending eastward to the plains.

Two patients sit in wheelchairs close to the large TV, its volume turned down. Magazines, paperbacks, and puzzles are scattered on tables and chairs. I wonder if they get newspapers, and which ones. I plan to spend a lot of time here getting the hell out of my room to drink coffee and read books. If there are no complaints from other patients, I may be able to watch football and hockey.

I am still basking in my proclamation when we arrive at a big room loaded with huge stainless steel tubs, lifts, and sinks. This is the area for bathing patients who cannot care for themselves. I am about to ask how frequently that occurs when a door opens beside me and I am forced to stand back as an extremely gaunt young man stumbles out of his room. His limbs are nearly without flesh, his skin loose over his bones. He has the appearance of being starved. Tubes run out of his nose and disappear down the frock that dangles from his tiny shoulders. He cannot walk without the aid of two nurses.

Shock must be glued to my face, because the nurse says, "Oh, don't worry; we can always feed you if you can't feed yourself." I continue to stare at the stricken man shuffling ahead until he is out of sight. She explains that he is back from home again, fighting the complications GVHD has caused his stomach.

The acronym stands for "graft-versus-host disease." This condition occurs when newly transplanted cells from the donor (called the graft) view the recipient's cells (called the host) as foreign and attack it. Various tissues and organs can be damaged, particularly the skin, liver, and digestive system. Chronic GVHD can last a lifetime and seriously impact a patient's health.

I do not recall my doctors identifying GVHD as a concern. Until now, I had assumed the result of my treatment would be either a healthy life or an untimely death. I had not contemplated the possibility of being severely debilitated after my transplant.

The man's appearance jars the confidence I was spouting about handling the effects of my treatment. But I have great doctors, the medical science is good, and I have an incredible donor. My outlook is further boosted by the incredible optimism, genuine concern, and touch of humor I sense from every staff member I meet as we walk the hallways. I am certain our rapport will be excellent, especially after they learn I expect to be roughed up by treatment, and have a plan to cope with the inevitable physical afflictions of life on Unit 57.

When I go off the trail while in the field, I always anticipate a degree of hardship. To meet it, I have cultivated a toughness

I call *hardiness.* The idols of my youth, the mountain men of the western frontier, were imbued with prodigious quantities of the stuff.

Hardiness is not complaining about the discomforts inherent in working outdoors. When you are thirsty, you wait to drink. Don't eat the moment you are hungry; wait until your hunger pangs subside. Whether you are short of breath, sweating profusely, wet to the skin, or shivering to the bone, you can train your mind to treat the situation as a nuisance, a temporary inconvenience—a condition you can remedy with patience.

Sufficient hardiness also creates a higher threshold for pain. I readily dismiss insect bites from mosquitoes, black flies, no-see-ums, horse and deer flies, gnats, sand flies, and ants. I can ignore the stings of bees, wasps, hornets, and nettles. Scrapes and bruises from falls, punctures from thorns, cuts from sharp grass, rashes from poisonous plants, and torn clothes are simply tolerable outcomes of a day in the field.

The entire process is one of restraint, a mind-over-matter dictum that began when I worked my first summer at a conservation camp in northern Wisconsin.

★ ★ ★ ★ ★

I was just finishing my sophomore year of high school (Grade 10), listening to the morning announcements in Miss Lewandowski's homeroom, when I heard of an opportunity to work in the field alongside professionals managing parks, forests, and fish and wildlife in Wisconsin. Six weeks, eighteen dollars a week, and every day outdoors in the land of my dreams, the Northwoods.

The camp, temporary home to nearly one hundred boys between sixteen and nineteen years old, was intimidating at first, especially when I was immediately afflicted with an acute case of homesickness. Camp discipline and routine, overseen in rigid military fashion by an ex-army colonel, soon became the perfect remedies for too much thinking of home.

Reveille was at 7:00 a.m.; we rode buses to work sites Monday through Friday. We returned to camp by 5:00 p.m. a half-hour before supper.

Free time occurred after supper, unless your large military-issue wall tent had scored the lowest on cleanliness and neatness during morning inspection. In that case, mundane tasks like painting, cutting grass, and shovelling gravel, supplemented with calisthenics and sprints, filled the evening hours. The tent with the lowest score for the week also worked Saturday afternoon which eliminated the weekend bus trip to the nearest town.

Our crew supervisors were typically strict and not beyond unusual punishments for misbehavior. One afternoon, my hard hat flew off when I popped my head up over the bed of our moving truck in response to, "Look at that chick!" After turning the truck around to retrieve my helmet, our boss pulled over and marched me into the hot and humid woods.

There I was ordered to strip. My bare feet felt strange touching the leaves and twigs on the forest floor as I fixed my arms by my sides. I had to stand at attention for ten minutes; if I was caught moving, my sentence would double.

The mosquitoes soon arrived for the immovable feast, able to land and suck to capacity without the danger of being crushed by slapping hands. I tried to blow them away from my face, only to expel more carbon dioxide that attracted more of the bloodthirsty insects. I was being attacked so heavily it was impossible to feel any one bite, but when I glanced down, my legs were peppered with mosquitoes while thick swarms looked for open spots to land.

I did not move. After getting my jeans and shirt back on, I reached for my socks while swatting the bugs off my feet. I counted seventeen bites just on the top of my right foot. I proudly announced this fact while receiving accolades from my crew mates for not being a sissy.

The following summer I returned to camp for both six-week sessions. I again wore my wounds like badges of honor, and developed a remarkable tolerance for being stung by yellow jackets and paper wasps. I was always on call to dispatch the nests we disturbed working in the woods, and enjoyed the reputation of toughness bestowed on me by the other boys.

★   ★   ★   ★   ★

My personal motto after decades in the field is: "tough nature brings out the best in a man." Why *tough* nature? It has been when experiencing the breath-taking forces of nature—thunderstorms, whiteouts, knock-down winds, big waves, fierce currents—that my spirit has truly become one with nature, and I have felt an endless energy and strength pervade my mind and body. It is not that I have the will to conquer nature (like a pioneer) but rather the ability to flow with the power of nature.

As my tour of Unit 57 concludes, I am convinced hardiness will help me focus my mind on healing and ward off the "fight or flight" moments that are bound to emerge in the months ahead. Maybe I can avoid the debilitating surges of adrenaline screaming *put up your fists* or *run, run faster*. I want to conserve my mental and physical resources as I would during a long expedition.

I thank the nurse for the tour. Tomorrow will be my last day of freedom.

★   ★   ★   ★   ★

Prior to admittance, my wife, daughters and I go for ice cream, and I ask to stop to look at the mallards we have noticed sitting in the snow along the road beside the walking path along the river. They are content to stay only a few feet from the trail, rarely moving unless a dog or a child walks into their midst.

The ducks are black in the whitish glare of the sun. I look away, spotting a pair standing alone on fresh ice at the river's edge. The plumage of the hen is richly textured, back-lit by the sun, and I stare at the orange legs of the drake, certain they will break through the shiny skim of ice.

People feed the ducks or they would not survive the months ahead.

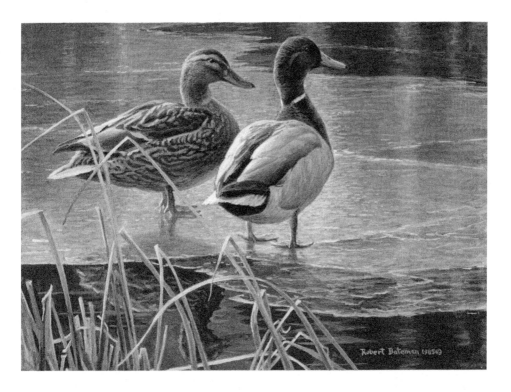

Mallard Pair-Early Winter

Chapter 10
Unit 57

You must never confuse faith that you will prevail
in the end—which you can never afford to lose—
with the discipline to confront the most brutal facts
of your current reality, whatever that might be.

–US Vice Admiral James Stockdale, quoted in *Good to*
Great by Jim Collins

My room is Spartan by choice. There is no phone to disrupt
my rest, and no TV—I can watch television in the lounge. The
Super Bowl is only a week away, and friends have promised to
visit me for the game.

I have a window in my room. Pigeons prance along the sill. I
have never found these birds interesting—their gaudy plumage
is bizarre, and they are no longer truly wild birds. They are an
introduced species, their ancestors arriving from Europe many
decades ago.

Perhaps I can change my attitude, enjoy their activity (if
I get bored), and use them as a link to the outside world I
will be prohibited from enjoying during the critical phases of
my treatment. At least pigeons are good food for hawks, owls,
and peregrine falcons. Maybe I will see one of these predators swoop down and pick one off. That would be something
worth watching for.

I have a fresh notebook to record my journey in Unit 57. Taking note of my travels is habitual: back home, journals from my field studies crowd the shelves in my office and are packed in boxes and stacked in the closet. Most of the daily entries start with the weather: temperature, wind speed and direction, cloud type and percent cover, precipitation, and storm activity. Then I start to compile data, usually sightings of animals, adding notes throughout the day about the blooming of plants and recent changes in the landscape. Before I leave the field, I recap my results and observations, noting my expectations of my next time afield. Closing the book has always been a satisfying conclusion to the proceedings of the day.

Now I will be the subject of my own field notes. No one will say how long I will be here, so I try to avoid any thoughts of leaving, escaping into the details of the procedures ahead, hoping to focus on the daily events of my treatment.

★ ★ ★ ★ ★

27 January. My first night in a hospital since that night in grade six when I broke my arm.

It was during recess on a blustery winter day and we were playing "tackle the bum." The game was simple, and any number of boys could play. The goal was to run with the ball, hat, glove or scarf in any direction, until you slipped, tripped, or were felled by a tackle, after which you were buried on the ground under a mound of bodies. It was gang tackling with no penalties for piling on despite the cries of "Get off, I can't breathe!" from the bottom of the heap.

I was pinned to the hard snow beneath a mass of boys with my left arm trapped, my elbow straight up and my hand bent topside down. The pain was building, my breath almost gone, when I felt the pop, my wrist snapping in two places. Clutching my arm to my chest, I tried not to cry until the nun supervising the playground led me inside. The game went on merrily without me.

If we had been allowed to play "king of the hill" on top of the giant piles of snow that surrounded the playground, I would not have been hurt. The teachers, however, were tired of sending us to the boys' room to sit on the radiators to dry off our pants.

My dad had the car at work, so a neighbor took me to the hospital. When the x-rays indicated a broken arm, it was too late to go home, so I was kept overnight.

For this stay, I have brought three of my favorite books, old, worn companions that have helped me weather storms in the past: *A Sand County Almanac* by Aldo Leopold to remind me of the beauty and harmony of nature; the copy of *Desert Solitaire* I had in camp when I was counting songbirds; and Peter Matthiessen's *The Snow Leopard,* to help me remain in the moment. Good reading to keep me close to my many loves of nature.

Last week, in another part of the hospital, Kathy had done her part after being delayed for hours by a blizzard in Minneapolis (arriving at 2:00 a.m. with nobody to greet her at the airport). She also got trapped in an elevator with our sister Carol on the day of stem cell collection.

Initially she had been given a drug called a colony-stimulating factor, which caused her blood stem cells to proliferate rapidly. After five days, "daughter cells" flooded her bloodstream. They were spun out by a machine while the other blood cells were returned to her body (she felt so well she went home the next day). Thus, the marrow cells I am to receive were not collected by needles inserted into Kathy's hip (the traditional process known to most people), but were gathered directly from the blood circulating around her body.

The technique is known as a peripheral stem cell transplant.

I will receive the stem cells through a vein, the same way as a blood transfusion. After infusion into my bloodstream, the transplanted stem cells will migrate to my clean bone marrow, where they will hopefully settle and start making new blood cells. Engraftment usually occurs within ten days to four weeks. Thereafter, if I survive, it will be one to two years before I have a fully functioning immune system stamped with Kathy's trademark.

28 January. The start of chemotherapy with fludarabine, the heaviest hitter of my drug protocol.

29 January. My sleep has been ragged the past two nights. I always sleep on my left side. Now, hooked up to a plethora of short tubes and wires either held by clamps to my pajamas or pasted to my shaved skin, I must lie on my back, tightly tethered to an IV and heart monitor. I am warned not to toss around in bed or I risk tearing out the central line that drips chemicals directly into my heart.

My room is noisy: the intercom above my head is never turned off, not even in the middle of the night. I can hear background noises through the static and learn to distinguish the clunk of a coffee cup from the thud of a thick manila folder. The various sounds at the front desk are soon more distinct than the songs of the closely related sparrows I have studied in the field.

And it is never truly dark. Even though there is a night-light nearby, the nurses insist on keeping my door open at least a few feet. I am scolded when I slink out of bed to close it. I tell them the spectrum of colored lights of the various monitors and devices in my room, winking and flashing throughout the night, can easily guide me to the bathroom. But I am told, "What if you fall and call for help? How will we hear you?"

I think of friends who have never spent a night alone. Because I have spent so much time overnight in the wilderness, I am used to things that go bump in the night. I wonder how many of the patients on Unit 57 are awake, hearing strange sounds, unable to sleep, and feeling scared. Staring at the dark, seeing shapes, wanting to flee somewhere safe.

30 January. It is a nuisance to go anywhere with my iron friend (the bedside IV pole hung with a bag of fluids that attach to my central line) but I walk along the corridors and do loops around the nursing station to maintain my strength. I never fail to happily say hello to the other patients walking the floor with their metal companions. We share stories of who we are, the details of our treatments, and our hopes for recovery.

Later in the day I watch the Super Bowl with my friend Shane. Even though the Packers aren't playing, it's a good game. The St. Louis Rams win.

31 January. The delivery of the various drugs I am to receive has begun in earnest. One of them gives me hallucinations; much of the previous night I spent with a chair floating through the room and a picture changing shapes as it glided across the wall.

It is only a small comfort when I am told, "We did that to you."

I get the shakes due to an unexpected allergic reaction to Demerol. A drug known as rabbit juice (because it is produced in bunnies) also gives me tremors, and I slip in the shower. My belief in hardiness sustains me.

A triple-sized desktop calendar has been taped on the wall of my room to record my blood counts, primarily my WBC. Fludarabine has beaten down my lymphocytes from 89,400 to 20,400 in only three days. The measurements are converted to 89.4 and 20.4. I must reach 1.5 or less before the cancer roaming my body is considered sufficiently destroyed, and my bone marrow is clean and ready for the transplant.

I love the calendar. It allows me to track the daily progress of my treatment, as if I were measuring the consecutive strides of a cougar moving ahead of me in the snow. Seeing the changes in the number of my cells feeds my well-being, suiting my analytic approach to recovery. The numbers are real, no longer an abstract notion of what is going on in my body.

The calendar is my only tangible lifeline to the future.

1 February. Each morning I change into jeans and a loose-fitting shirt because I want to feel normal. However, as the drugs suppress my immune system, hairs from my head begin to stick to my pillow. I am not perturbed. Without hair, I can avoid haircuts, which I have endured with anxiety throughout my life, stigmatized from childhood until senior high by the brush-cuts enforced by my dad.

My classmates called me Lightbulb or Light, given the shape of my head. When my zips grew bristly between cuts, my closest friends called me Hedgehog or Hedge. At least I had nicknames fondly given, ones that I enjoyed.

My wife gives me a Bozo haircut to bring some humor to the floor. The next day, the rest is cut. I feel good. Baldness in men is becoming fashionable. It's a look I associate with being a bad-ass.

2 February. My seventh day on the ward. Despite my change in appearance, and the sterile surroundings, my wife and I do not discuss our feelings. Personal thoughts about the future have been hidden for so long, it is tough to put them on the table even when our situation is real, immediate, and possibly deadly. Instead, we play cribbage and talk about our children.

WBC falling fast: 8.8. I am anxious to receive Kathy's donor cells (which are sitting in a fridge somewhere). The preparatory drugs are making me jittery and light-headed, and I am losing my appetite.

I do not read my books or write much; anxiety overpowers my concentration after a few sentences. When the pigeons characteristically jerk their heads while walking by, I get dizzy. I look beyond them to a small section of trees along the Bow River, a slice of nature in the distance. Mostly spruce, maybe a few fir trees on the driest sites. I know there are big poplars below, but I cannot see them.

3 February. My WBC has dropped steeply overnight to 1.4. The big yellow smiley face drawn on my calendar announces "Happy Transplant Day."

My sister is a loyal fan of the Green Bay Packers, a diehard, and we have decided to use football as an analogy for the events of this special day (the arrival of her daughter marrow cells). Our scene unfolds like this:

It is late afternoon on the frozen tundra at Lambeau Field. The Super Bowl. We have been playing hard, underdogs, hurting from the hits we have taken, our uniforms and helmets muddy and cold. We are driving for the winning score, the championship, but are only at midfield.

The clock is running out as we line up, our breath curling away into the stadium lights, the fans on their feet. Kathy nods at me and drops back, ducking a linebacker and rolling right to avoid tacklers as she looks for me streaking down the sidelines. She unloads the ball as she is hit, a perfect spiral arching high over the field. Running between defenders, I dive to catch the pass, tumbling into the end zone. Touchdown! The crowd roars in disbelief. The gun sounds. We win!

Now that I have made the grab, it is Day 0, and we start a new tally, a drive to 100 days, the milestone that means I have survived the most vulnerable period of my recovery. But first Kathy's cells must accept my body and settle into my bones, and quickly produce new infection-fighting cells in my marrow.

I am told to expect the joy of scoring to be short-lived. Patients routinely hit the wall physically by Day 2 because their bodies have been faltering under the cumulative impact of the conditioning chemotherapy. Soon thereafter, the major organs, including the skin, which I have never thought of as an organ, can be severely weakened or damaged, and bodily functions typically run off the tracks.

That will be the time to summon maximum hardiness.

Day 2. Still holding my own and able to leave my room. I like to stop at the bulletin board where a postcard showing a former patient standing poolside, somewhere warm, always deserves another look. He is healthy and has hair, and I am certain the plastic cup in his hand holds beer. He is alive and well, and I smile at him. I plan to post a photo of me too when I am well—hopefully one from a tropical paradise.

A man comes to visit the patient in the room beside me. I see that he usually stands in the hallway, head down, back against the wall for several minutes before he walks into the room. We never speak, but simply acknowledge each other with a nod. I usually stand by the wall, too, hoping he will find comfort in my simple presence and apparent good health. I never learn his name.

My wife visits every day, commuting from our friend's condo on the far south side of Calgary. I can see she is weary from the drive and the days alone in the city. I encourage her to go home to rejoin our daughters (Alysia is home from New York watching her younger sisters), insisting I can manage by myself.

Day 4. A visiting doctor from England makes the rounds instead of my usual one. I am admiring my chart, sitting by the window (still waiting for a pigeon to die).

He smiles, noting that my skin is as red as a cooked lobster. I assure him it is just a touch of GVHD, no more painful than a mild sunburn, despite some blisters.

He asks me to grip and squeeze his hands, the usual test for monitoring my strength. He is surprised at the power I have in my hands. When he asks me why I am not using a morphine pump, I shrug. I say I don't need one, although the sores along my gums are starting to fester.

I want to tell him about my philosophy of hardiness but before I can explain, he looks up from his chart and says, "Mr. Herzog, you are one tough son of a bitch."

Tougher than nails, I think, as he leaves the room. I am three days beyond the normal point of crashing: I might just get by without the usual suffering.

Day 5. My skin burns hotter with GVHD and I grimace at the touch of my sheets. Hardiness helps me endure the pain but fails when my scrotum feels like it is lit on fire. I am told not to put ice directly on my burning balls (directions I quickly ignore). One of the nurses adds, "We did that to you, too," grinning as she leaves my room.

Later in the day, I try to take a shower. The gentlest stream of water burns my entire body. I dare not dry my skin with a towel.

I try to eat soft foods, but even pudding spikes the pain in my mouth. I cannot squeeze any saliva from my cheeks, so the bread I finally swallow scours my throat. My taste buds are shot, and the smell of any warm food makes my stomach turn.

I do not dress in street clothes today.

Day 6. I sit hunched over my tray, a queasy feeling churning in my stomach. I gag down meager pieces of shredded chicken after washing off the nauseating teriyaki sauce, knowing I must eat protein because it is essential to the growth of my budding immune system. I doubt I can force-feed myself much longer; luckily, I like the taste of Ensure and other high-protein drinks (except for anything strawberry-flavored) and soon abandon solid food.

That night I am suddenly ablaze and drenched in sweat. Soon I am freezing and shaking from cold. My sheets are tossed on the floor and I am buried under heated blankets, but I later kick them off the bed.

A code goes out over the intercom. I never know what color. Hot, cold, hot, cold. Nurses stay by my side throughout the endless night.

They say I am talking gibberish.

Day 7. When I am lucid during the day, I focus on the distant patch of evergreens I had seen earlier from my window. Big spruce trail up the slope to a cliff where houses perch above the rocks. The trees are ideal habitat for red squirrels. They are feisty little creatures, packing both energy and attitude in their compact bodies, especially when defending their hoards of cones and seeds. They are always aware of danger and scold intruders vociferously, barking, chattering, and screeching while stamping their feet, alerting everyone in the forest. Being at the bottom of the food chain has made them wary.

That evening, the fever returns. I squeeze my eyes tight, and in my mind, I am trying to sneak by the squirrels without being seen. I imagine a bright winter day, late afternoon. I walk only a few steps at a time, the falling sun at my back, long angles of light piercing the snowy edge of the forest. I crouch against one of the biggest trees, kneeling on the dry ground in the smooth bowl of wind-swept snow spun around its trunk, my hand touching the rough, sticky bark. Still no alarm. I creep to my next lookout, peering into the shadowy interior of the woods ahead.

I also try to recall exactly where and how I had seen poisonous snakes on the trail to the macaws, or think about being in the wintry mountains, tracking a moose or lynx, my pants getting wet as I flounder in the deep snow.

Sometimes the memories are astoundingly vivid. If I can focus on the fine details of a scene, it feels likes it is really happening. When this occurs, I can dispel the worry and suffering of the night for several soothing moments. Nonetheless, I am using my last ounces of hardiness, rapping on the glass in the daytime to scare the pigeons away, running on empty.

Days 8-11. I dread the arrival of the searing routine of burning and freezing that now comes every night within a few fearful minutes of 7:10 p.m. I wish it were only malaria—at least then the fever that lasts for hours would have a cause.

Each night, the same technician arrives to draw blood. She tries to disguise the troubled look on her face, but I overhear her telling the nurses rotating my blankets that the cultures keep coming back empty.

I am in danger, but do not think of dying. Months later, I find out how close I was to the edge (the doctors didn't know what was happening, and with no identifiable cause, they were at a loss at how to treat me).

Although I don't know it, my situation now is more precarious than when I waded one black morning with crocodiles.

★ ★ ★ ★ ★ ★

Wild storms tearing limbs from the trees had kept all of us indoors. Heavy rain lashed the metal roof over our heads night and day: none of us could be heard over the din without shouting. Thunderous lightning had knocked out the power and the cook had not come to work for three days. There were no eggs and we were tired of eating rice and beans.

I awoke an hour earlier than usual. The forest was dripping, but the rain had stopped sometime in the night. Forgetting my machete, I hurried to my bike, confident that the mice and snakes had headed for higher ground.

The potholes were brimming with rainwater and soon I was raising my feet to the handlebars. After nearly falling in one of the deeper pools and losing my headlamp, I abandoned the bike, sloshing ahead.

My boots, filled with the muddy water, became anchors. Soon the water was flowing to my knees—I would never reach the lookout by dawn to count the macaws. Yet another delay in collecting the data.

Only then did I think about the crocodiles living along the river.

Might they have followed the floodwaters inland? Where was that beast I had seen trolling up the river last week? That piece of yellow plastic in its teeth was the ear tag of a young beef cow about my size.

My headlamp was gone, but I still had my flashlight; its light bounced off water swirling with debris. I could not see any eyes reflected in the beam, but would I before being dragged under? Guns were prohibited in the national park, and without my machete I was defenseless. I grabbed a floating stick. Should I put my pocket-knife between my teeth?

The water was at my waist. I thought of turning back, but I thought I saw the hazy outline of the observation hill ahead. Propelled by the scientific rigor that demands all surveys be done in identical fashion, I plunged ahead. At times like this, the discipline to collect good data requires a stiff measure of craziness.

I started breathing again when I reached the safety of the hill. The sense of danger eased momentarily until I thought of stranded snakes (or anything else that might bite).

The macaws were wet and subdued when they flew by, and I did not hear the call of monkeys. Nor were there any vultures overhead in the rain-laden clouds.

After several hours, the floodwaters receded, so it was safe to trek back to the ranger station. The deluge began again before I could park my bike.

★ ★ ★ ★ ★ ★

Day 12. After a week of agony, the fevers mysteriously stop. The danger is past, but I am crushed by an avalanche of fatigue. The nurses help me get out of bed for the morning weigh-in, standing alongside me so I do not fall. I cannot take a bath alone and I am astonished that I must sit to pee, my bladder unable to generate more than a slow drip.

I shamble about my room, barely able to stay upright and out of bed. I do not want to eat or drink. I am debilitated and decimated by my ordeal. How could I have been so naive and stupid to think I could skate by unscathed while other patients suffered so greatly?

My WBC has been hovering at 0.4 for the past week—there is no sign of engraftment.

Day 14. Late in the day I sit in a wheelchair by the pay phone at the far end of the hallway. I decide to call my parents. Home.

When I hear my mom's voice, I start to cry. I need to console and be consoled.

My mom's cancer is worsening and I don't want to add to their worries, so I give my parents a positive report.

After we talk, I decide I don't want my conversation with them to have been only false bravado. I can do better to get well. But things are so hard.

Day 17. When the nurse comes into my room, she is hiding a smile. She blocks the calendar, knowing I can read the numbers from my bed. As she stands aside, a huge yellow sun edged with orange exclaims 0.8!

Kathy's donor cells *are* settling into my bone marrow. We exchange high-fives and I receive congratulations from staff throughout the day. But, strangely, I am not overjoyed. I am so sick. I do not even call Kathy to thank her for saving my life.

Day 19. The nights of fever have rocked me, and I am much diminished in body, mind and spirit since the start of that ordeal. I struggle to regain any degree of optimism.

The side effects of treatment continue to worsen. I do not care to eat and the nurses must remind me to drink. The chemo has parboiled me on the outside and microwaved me on the inside, and I fear a return of the fevers.

My blood counts have improved (my WBC printout reads 4.0) but I am unable to study them for inspiration. I am so, so tired.

I cannot read and rarely write; words and letters are mired in a maze, and although I have nothing to do, I do not think of leaving my room. I never ask about the time of day.

I can no longer visualize the red squirrels, the shiny mallards that sit on the ice along the river (perhaps they have died), or the jackrabbits outside the hospital making tracks in the snow. I no longer think of nature.

I am lost, becoming a stranger in my own mind. I must have fumbled the ball before I got in the end zone. A counselor talks to me about depression.

Day 21. I am shocked when I'm switched to a double room. I believed I would never leave *my* room until I was going home. It has been my safe place, my refuge against fears of failure.

Although the move means I am making progress, it is a sharp blow to my confidence.

My roommate only returns at night, free on day passes. He runs his TV loud, so I withdraw into myself, hoping to silence the noise that invades my space from the other side of the curtain.

Day 25. I move to another room with a man who refuses to talk to me although we need to share a bathroom. He wears the same torn, stained Minnesota Vikings sweatshirt—a team that hates the Packers—every day. Its sleeves are cut off in wife-beater fashion. He frequently curses the nurses, initially prompting visits by senior staff. When his foul-mouthed rants continue, a security guard arrives, sitting outside our room for hours.

I keep quiet, focusing my thoughts on the texture of the beige paint on the wall, the occasional dust bunny on the floor, and the joints in the drop-down ceiling. I loosely mark time by the arrival of meals I do not want, and the start of darkness outside my window. Somehow both time and space are compressed, the air tight and stale.

I am fearful of leaving my room. I have withdrawn inward.

Day 28: The old brick of the adjacent building blocks my view of the river valley. It doesn't matter; I no longer care what is happening in the natural world.

Day 33: I am startled when the nurses rush in and start packing my clothes, taking my once-beloved chart off the wall, helping me to get dressed. Somehow, some way, I am too well to be in the hospital. No one has told me I was going anywhere. It is all too soon, too sudden. I am prodded to move.

I do not want to leave, but I do not complain, feigning happiness. I am in a daze, disembodied, and do not read the papers on my lap indicating I am being "discharged in stable condition with discharge medications of prednisone [anti-GVHD], cyclosporine [anti-rejection] and Septra [anti-infection]. Patient to monitor his temperature several times a day and call Unit 57 immediately if above 100°F."

I am wheeled to the waiting car, blinded by the sun.

Chapter 11
Home

Being ill is a perpetual balancing of faith and will.

—Arthur W. Frank, *At the Will of the Body:*
Reflections on Illness

I only travel a few miles to my friend Richard's condo because I must stay in town until I clear the danger zone for infections and outbursts of GVHD. My anxiety lessens when I realize help is only a phone call away and that my daughters will be arriving for the weekend.

We have a belated party to celebrate Katie's 12th birthday, and visitors arrive from Lethbridge and Wisconsin. I receive a Packer toque which I wear to capture the heat leaving my bald head. Regular trips to the outpatient clinic show good clinical results despite low neutrophil counts and a moderate case of liver GVHD. I tell no one, but I remain as detached from my surroundings as I had on Unit 57.

On Day 77, I am on my way home after six weeks at the condo. Yesterday I was disappointed when I learned I had to return to the hospital in three weeks: I cannot recall ever being told I would be undergoing radiation on my groin.

Arriving at home is not the celebration I had gleefully anticipated before I left for treatment. The place looks the same and I receive a cheerful welcome from my daughters, but it does not feel like home. The space is wrong, unsettling. The rooms are altered in some strange way, and the hallways lead to unfamiliar places. I walk cautiously, feeling trapped and uneasy, on edge. The entire environment is odd and, sadly, without comfort.

I am alone every day when my wife is at work and the girls are at school. I had anticipated enjoying the quiet time to watch TV and read magazines, novels, and all my recent wild-life journals. I planned to indulge myself by leisurely searching the web without feeling guilty about the loss of time.

But I do not use a computer.

I do not read.

I do not watch TV.

There is too much color, too much action on the screen. The stories are too complex or unfold too quickly. I plug my ears at the first sounds of mildly harsh language and weep openly at the mere suggestion of violence. If a scene anticipates a car accident, even if someone is clearly walking safely across the street, I visualize myself being killed by a car. I do not want to go outside.

When I try to read, I lose the meaning of the story after a few paragraphs, missing important details. When I reread the sentences with renewed concentration, my thoughts are over-powered by the effort, further muddling my understanding.

When I try to write, my pen stops after a few words. When I continue, I scribble, as my hand cannot travel fast enough to record my thoughts. Anyone could forge my checks; I cannot complete my own signature.

When I try to use the computer, the keyboard is too complex. I cannot control the mouse and its rapid motion is so abrupt, it distorts my vision.

I do not listen to the news. The media coverage is skewed to disasters, wars, and human suffering. Doomsday events domi-nate predictions of the future.

I do not listen to music. It never occurs to me to do so.

When I do go outside, hoping to enjoy the early days of spring, I must wear a mask to ward off spores and pollen and cannot go near plowed earth, cut grass, and compost (where there might be fungi and bacteria that could kill me). I may have to live indoors forever, disconnected from nature.

What do I do?

On the living room wall is a large batik of an elephant and an antelope I bought while working in Africa. The two animals are standing beside a narrow orange and black carrot-topped tree. The elephant is also black and orange, its legs strangely too long for its body. It covers half the scene. The antelope is a rosy tone, grazing on a low green wave of grass. It is the same size as the elephant, a recurring mystery I try to unravel.

The animals absorb my attention for hours each day as I wait aimlessly for people to come home. I always concentrate on the under-sized ear of the elephant, and wait for the hues of colors to shift gradually at dusk. I do not think, but I am aware, the animals a barrier to intruding thoughts. I imagine I have a blank look on my face.

My radiation treatments start next week. I insist I can drive myself to Calgary, where I will stay alone at Richard's place. This is my chance to start living again, to have days with a sense of purpose.

I will be able to watch wildlife from the condo: deer are attracted to the yard, feeding on shrunken apples, some of which still cling to the branches of the tree. A pellet gun stands by the patio doors—I have promised to discourage the squirrels from raiding the bird feeders while Richard is in Africa.

★ ★ ★ ★ ★

When I arrive at the condo, there is no fresh food. I boldly trek the few blocks to the nearby store, the farthest distance

I have walked since the transplant. The sun feels good on my face and neck, and I see myself walking the trails in the nearby river valley.

I am immediately discouraged. Returning from the store, I am unsteady and start weaving into the soccer field beside the road. Then I am on my knees—fruit, bread, and canned goods spilled on the thawing ground.

A blue jay cries and I hear tires crunching gravel on the nearest road.

Two young boys watch me from the sidewalk where they are packing icy snowballs. I call them over.

"Can you help me pick up my groceries?"

"Yeah, we can, but do you want me to go get our mom?"

"No, it's fine," I say. "If you could carry my bags to the street corner, I can manage from there. It's just a short block to my place."

Once inside, I go directly to bed.

Traffic is heavy the second morning I leave for the hospital. When I pull away from a green light, mucous and small pieces of food flow uncontrolled from my mouth onto the front of my shirt. The episode repeats itself without burping, heaving or nausea. I return to the condo.

I take a cab to the hospital the next day. Neither the radiologists nor the doctors at the outpatient clinic can explain why I have no control over the upper end of my system.

I am instructed to try digestive enzymes, the theory being my stomach is affected by the radiation. They do not work and my predicament worsens when I have diarrhea. I am careful to scout the location of every men's room along the hallways of the radiation floor, but need to roll out extreme hardiness to tightly squeeze my butt cheeks while launching myself onto and off the radiation treatment table—I do not want to have an accident while lying there. I start to wear diapers day and night.

Determined to keep pushing upslope, I struggle to complete the final rounds of radiation. Cab drivers are leery of the ice cream pail on my lap, but I am too weak to drive.

Day 100 arrives, an incredibly important milestone. By surviving this far, I have beaten the odds, and my chances of gaining remission are improving daily.

But there is no excitement, because I'm told I must postpone my final two sessions. I finally complete them and hole up at the condo, waiting for a ride home.

★ ★ ★ ★ ★

A crow hops along the shoulder of the road, flapping its wings. There is a ruddy patch on the road nearby where a large animal has been hit: there must be roadkill in the ditch, hidden by the tall, dull winter grass.

A sharp wind pulls tears from my eyes as I inhale the cold air, hoping to quell the queasiness rolling up my throat. The trip home has become a brutal test of endurance, the speed and motion of highway travel rocking my equilibrium. I feel as if cars and trucks are hurtling toward me: I flinch when they go by in the opposite lane. Road signs threaten to smash into us. If I close my eyes, I only feel more vulnerable, anticipating a crash in the darkness.

At home the nausea subsides, but am I besieged with immense urges to go. I swallow handfuls of stool softeners, and gulp laxatives and magnesium citrate, but my bowels refuse to move. The twice-daily enemas I give myself while lying exhausted on the bathroom floor are sadly ineffective. After an agonizing ten days, I start retching at night and am ordered back to Unit 57.

Crying from the cramps, I spend the trip gasping and straining perched atop a makeshift port-a-potty (a tall white plastic bucket that once held construction glue), my head against the ceiling of the van. An aide meets us at the entrance to the cancer centre and pushes me into the elevator in a wheelchair, an empty ice cream bucket again on my knees.

After receiving an IV (I am severely dehydrated), I am rushed to the x-ray department for a picture of my abdomen. My intestinal tract is completely blocked from top to bottom. A colonoscopy is booked for two days hence. In preparation, I start drinking a sweet orange syrup (lactulose), and the following day, I stagger frequently to the bathroom, barely able to control the volcanic reactions erupting from my lower quadrant.

I am awake at the start of the exam and invited by the doctor to follow the procedure on the TV screen. Once I understand his comments, I see the severe lesions in my intestinal tract. It is one of the few times I wish I were not a biologist who knows what he is looking at. I am offered a close-up color snapshot of the results when I meet the doctor the next day.

The stomach and intestinal problems I have endured over the past month are the delayed results of chemotherapy.

The staff assure me I will be feeling better soon (my system improves with hydration and prednisone), and I begin to nibble at solid food. I renew my walks around the ward, but do not see the quiet man who previously stood in the hallway beside my old room. Hopefully whomever he was visiting is home and doing well.

The familiar surroundings improve my mood. After all, I am not back because of GVHD or a return of the cancer. One of my nurses tells me she could have made money showing my stomach x-ray throughout the hospital. Everyone is amazed how full of "it" I had been. I feel special in a funny sort of way, and I enjoy the feelings of camaraderie that continue in the following days. I admire the way the nurses and staff hustle through the ward, and I have yet to hear harsh words between them.

After being allowed to sit downstairs in the common area on the main floor, I beg to walk outside. I promise to stay on the hospital grounds (I am too weak to go far, anyway).

I cheat by walking across the street to the sidewalk that runs beside a small patch of poplar trees. I'm wearing my hospital gown—maybe someone in the cars passing by will report me as a runaway.

All the trees high on the slope have gnarly crowns. Hmm . . . seems like I have never noticed that before. I see some shrubs in the undergrowth but do not recognize them (I should know what species they are at a glance). A path runs through the grass.

I spot a small woodpecker making the rounds of the bigger trees. I try to identify the bird, but I am not even sure what characteristics to look for. This is wacky; I know how to tell the little woodpeckers apart with a quick glimpse. I think of approaching the bird, but the ground is muddy.

My discharge is imminent after two weeks. Now that I am improving, I believe there is little chance I will ever return to the unit, so before I leave, I decide to visit my old room a final time. The intercom blares "Code Blue!" and staff race ahead of me.

There is a man slumped on the floor, face in his hands. When he glances my way, I recognize him—he is the one who stood in the hallway near my door. I slide down the wall a few feet away from him, my legs out, and I am sobbing instantly.

Whom has he loved so deeply and lost after all the weeks of hope? A wife, a mom, a sister, a brother? I had never asked the name of the person he came to see.

A few days later, at home, I am compelled to find words for a rough poem.

Unit 57 – The Cancer Ward

Shackled inside is a spirit searching for light,
Unable to sense the eerie surroundings with all its might.

Mortal fear of dying is always near,
Pain and suffering everywhere to see and hear.

Why fight when the bargain is struck,
Can survival be anything more than simple luck?

Each breath and thought must become its own reward,
Or it becomes hopeless in the turmoil of the cancer ward.

Sleep is never peaceful, so often startled by shouts of
"Code Blue,"
You feel guilty when you pray that the next time won't
be you.

Tears and worry each hour come anew,
Faces of patients change daily, possessions are few.

Name tags are replaced often outside many a room,
Life or death disappears before staff enters with mop
and broom.

But faith and will are rebuilt most by those that leave,
And later return intact, therefore no need to grieve.

Chapter 12

Fear of Living

No one argued I was officially recovering. No one knew that I had somehow taken a psychologically dark turn inside. I was losing hope.

—Wayson Choy, *Not Yet: A Memoir of Living and Almost Dying*

I soon miss the daily banter I shared with my nurses and doctors. I also miss their constant encouragement on my progress, however slim, and the human touch so simply received by the stacking of pillows or a fresh glass of water. I miss the warm blankets: I am always cold and can no longer thermoregulate. I feel like an amphibian.

I even miss the occasional scolding for forgetting to rinse my teeth. And how I always feigned anger when the nurses' response to some new problem with my body was met by, "Oh, don't worry, we did that to you," while secretly I was relieved the cause was known.

Now I have no one to ask about the problems assaulting me.

I feel a wave of dizziness when I lift my head off the pillow in the morning. Everything seems distant and moving just beyond my mental reach. My thinking seems to be getting more twisted and foggier, yet my mind never ceases to buzz with the noise of random thoughts. I am too stimulated or overtired to enjoy the seduction and pleasure of naps on the couch. When I wake at night, I am startled to realize I was never drowsy before falling asleep.

The mysterious stomach-bowel problem eventually disappears, but eating is a chore. Lettuce sticks in my throat and eating bread is like chewing cardboard. I choke when I try to wash it down with milk or water. Soup burns my mouth before I can register its temperature. Apples are too crisp and carrots are too hard. Grapefruit is prohibited because it affects the potency of my medications, especially the anti-rejection drugs critical to my recovery.

Shane brings me a Boston cream doughnut from Tim Horton's. They are my favorite Tim's treat. Today, even a small bite is too much. It's more sugar than I have eaten in weeks.

My taste buds are missing in action: the only food that has an authentic taste is peanut butter. I eat it plain, from the edge of a spoon, swishing it around in my mouth, licking it off my teeth. I am addicted to its magical, earthy flavor. I subsist on it, juice, protein drinks, pudding and ice cream.

I did not foresee having nothing to do, no one to call. I did not anticipate my home would be a no-man's land. I did not think it would be hard to see the big picture—that I could have been dead by now.

I decide to try driving again: Canada geese will be nesting at Henderson Lake, the big city park a few miles away. I soon lose confidence, braking suddenly to avoid hitting the cars stopped at intersections. I see them, but I react in slow motion, my foot failing to move unless a collision is imminent. Part of my pre-transplant protocol was an eye exam to detect the possible growth of cataracts—maybe my eyes are starting to cloud over. I adapt by driving below the speed limit, but feel endangered by the flow of the angry traffic dodging around me.

I also suffer from tunnel vision, not trusting my mirrors, hesitating to change lanes or turn into oncoming traffic, and second-guessing the overhead signs at intersections directing drivers to the correct turning lanes.

I am a threat to both drivers and pedestrians.

I quit driving.

These troubles are soon mimicked outdoors. My spatial awareness, always so acute while in the field, is gone. I am wobbly on the trails, pushed sideways as if by a hard wind. I have no peripheral vision, jump at shadows, and trip on branches that have fallen across the path. I see neither the forest nor the trees.

How will I ever walk along a mountain ridge, jump on rocks to cross a rushing stream, or scoot uphill? How will I wade through the muck of a cattail marsh when I can barely walk on uneven ground? I feel unsafe, as if the bears I feared as a child are chasing me.

I have no remedy for my disorientation. I only detect my strange reactions to my surroundings after they occur, and I cannot anticipate them beforehand. It is a bizarre situation; my body and mind are somehow unnaturally disconnected from each other, whether I am inside or outside. I no longer have a nimble mind or body.

I now stay in bed most of the day. I no longer get dressed in the morning. Yet I attempt to be strong for those around me, rarely complaining about my predicament. I talk of fun things we'll soon be doing like planting the garden, going to the cabin in Wisconsin, and going to the mountains during the summer.

My wife remains distant and strangely preoccupied. When I try to talk to her about my fears, her response is, "You just have to do it." I assume she needs her own space and time to recover from the disruption my treatment has brought to her life and to our family. I become trapped in an intensifying spiral of worry and anxiety: if I do not get healthy soon, I will be a poor husband and father, a drain on my family.

As this sense of failure overwhelms me, an e-mail arrives: I have lost my position at the college. New duties, yet undetermined, will be assigned to me when I am well enough to return to work. I am now on long-term disability. My identity as a professor, researcher, and biologist is shattered.

My willingness to cope with each new predicament and problem is slipping. Graphic nightmares packed with blood and gore invade my sleep, and the relentless turmoil adds to my imprecise sense of reality. My only relief occurs when I am in the actual moment of falling onto the couch or bed: my despair returns as soon as my head touches the pillow.

I try to recover my sanity by recalling wildlife adventures, like I did on Unit 57. The images are blurry, and I am unable to maintain a logical sequence of events. What develops is a disjointed array of broken scenes like those of my nightly dreams, so I quit trying to visualize happy moments outdoors (or any others in my life).

I have only been rarely afraid of dying from cancer, but now I am deathly afraid of living. I cannot live crippled by treatment without the comfort of home, a sense of belonging, or the future possibility of being able to wait in the dark for wildlife. I am endangered, and for the first time ever, I feel like a cancer *victim*. I have survived so far, but when I try to think of a good life ahead, I can find nothing in the world I want to do, nowhere I want to go.

The African batik is again my only refuge. I am bewitched by the massive butterfly that floats above the antelope, one wing green, the other purple, but it is not enough. I have lost my last remnants of hope, and am on the fine edge of losing my last shreds of faith. It is too hard to be strong.

I think about the guns in my closet. I debate loading them, each time closer to being unable to see an alternative.

I look at the phone, my hotline to Unit 57. I watch it for several minutes, thoughts of ending my life taking clearer shape.

Suicide is the solid choice I am being pulled toward. But then I realize the overpowering outcomes of unleashing that event.

Should I call the unit after everything they have done for me? I don't want to be a pest.

The nurse immediately recognizes my voice.

She asks, "Have you thought of hurting yourself?"

"Yes."

"Are there guns in the house?"

"Yes."

"Sit tight. Stay with me. Help is on the way."

Chapter 13
Hopeful

This evening I feel much better – why? I hate this black ravine; thick clouds are moving north, with threat of snow, and already the porters are pointing toward the pass, shaking their heads. Yet I feel calm, and ready to accept whatever comes, and therefore happy.

–Peter Matthiessen, *The Snow Leopard*

Another wheelchair, another appearance at Unit 57. I have been forced to return, and I hate the place. I have only been gone a month.

I sit on the edge of my bed, facing the wall. Head in my hands, broken. I have failed everyone. I have quit, and for the first time since all this began, I believe there is no one on Unit 57 who can help me.

Dr. Chaudhry immediately comes in and kneels in front of me. His posture surprises me because he is now the one who must look up to make eye contact. He tenderly grips my hands, and for a moment, we're held in silence.

"You have been my best patient ever," he says. "Your positive attitude has been a marvelous influence on both patients and staff. Yes, I know you do not want to be here, but you had been sick for a very long time, many years before you came to me. You have continued to be strong for months for those you love, but now, let me take care of you. You are in the best place you can be right now."

In that moment, I am no longer miles from nowhere.

He understands my desperation, my hopelessness about the future, and my feelings about having been left alone to survive. He visits me several times a day until I start walking the hallways.

At first, I am on suicide watch and cannot leave the ward. I don't mind the confinement because I am not alone. I listen to the sounds of activity outside my room, content to rest throughout the day. Sometimes I look out my window and try to track and count the cars using the parking ramp. I wonder how the attendants know if the lot is full.

When I start to make human contact by hanging quietly around the workstations, I realize I must be feeling better. Eventually, as I find myself sharing stories with other patients, I grow better in heart and soul. In some way, I find my thinking is sharper on Unit 57 than it is when I am at home. Certainly, the environment is more comforting than the surroundings of my house.

A young teenage boy becomes my roommate. He is in rough shape, being fed liquid through a nose tube. His mother sits in a chair by his side, never leaving the room. Toward evening, my nurse asks if the boy's mom can sleep overnight with him. I agree and have the best sleep I have had in weeks (maybe getting a share of the energy of motherly love floating in the room).

After two weeks, I have permission to leave the ward for short periods. I can sit downstairs in the patients' lobby. I am on the honor system to mind the time and not overstay my absence from the floor. By following the rules, I am finally allowed brief forays outdoors, where I sit, sheltered from the wind, across from the little woods where I last saw the wood-pecker I could not name. I like watching the trees.

My time allowed outside grows to half an hour, so one day I look for the bird. The hill, however, is much too steep to climb, so I abandon the search, preferring to sit above the long slope of short yellow grass that descends to the boundary of the cancer centre. I can see the trees along the river valley. The mallards of winter could now be nesting—there are little islands offshore, safe from predators.

I touch the grass, threading my fingers through the short stems. I take a few steps downhill, then a few more. It is the kind of hill ideal for tobogganing—one you could rocket down before crashing at high-speed.

My momentum carries me aimlessly to the bottom. I lie on the ground, the sun heating my back and legs. I melt as the solid earth pulls the tension from my body and relaxes my mind.

Perhaps I sleep, but suddenly I know I have been away from the ward too long and will be missed. When I start to climb, my knees buckle, and I sit, first for a few minutes, then for several more before I am on my hands and knees, crawling up the hill, pressing my face into the grass when I rest.

I wave to a man walking uphill on the sidewalk. He comes over to help me, and I lean heavily on him until we reach the front door of the hospital.

When I stumble off the elevator, the search party being organized to find me is disbanded, and my off-floor privileges are revoked until I am discharged the following week. At least I had been outside for a few moments, light-headed from the intoxicating smell and warmth of the spring air.

Chapter 14
Alone

The southbound tracks were noteworthy, not just because they were made by a tiger, but because there were large gaps—ten feet or more—between each set of impressions. At the point where they met, the northbound tracks disappeared, as if the person who made them had simply ceased to exist.

–John Valiant, *The Tiger: A True Story of Vengeance and Survival*

I return home for the fourth time, seven months since I first entered the hospital. My hands quiver and I am gaunt, bald, and thin. If I stood in a forest of saplings, no one could see me.

My weight is finally up a few pounds from the low of 124 I set during my last stay in the hospital. My pre-transplant weight had been 155 pounds, and when I look in the mirror now, the atrophy of my muscles is appalling; the loose and wrinkled skin flapping on my biceps especially disgusts me. It will be hard to gain weight—food still holds no taste (except for the unbelievable peanut butter). I try to eat a wide variety of salads and meats, but my salivary glands are too dry. Hunger will remain a thing of the past.

I am too weak for regular exercise, but enjoy walking while the girls ride their bikes ahead of me, happy to hear them laugh, recalling how I had once held their handlebars as they learned to pedal with small feet. I am too unstable to ride my bike, so I concentrate on moving smoothly, trying not to feel like an invalid.

Most of the time, I wander around the house and yard, needing to stay clear of the garden. I still go inside when my neighbor cuts the grass or when the wind is too strong.

Indoors we try playing cards, but I am too slow in recognizing suits and numbers. One of the girls checks my hand to make sure I am playing the right card and totals my points at the end of the game. These are simple games I taught my kids years ago, and now I am the one trying to learn the rules. Curiously, I am more amazed than discouraged by my ineptitude.

Too soon, it is time for school. My daughters return to class and my wife goes back to work as a teacher's aide.

The anti-depressant helps control my mood. I no longer think of suicide, but negative thoughts still appear sporadically. Dr. Chaudhry emphasized that I needed to be watchful and patient after the trauma of my earlier episode. Nothing can be worse than those black holes of crushing oblivion and despair, so I gently look after myself, careful to avoid expectations of the future. My brothers come to visit and bolster my spirits.

I feel best when I exist solely in the simplified environment of my home, free from schedules and deadlines, content with the well-wishes from my friends. I cope with my foggy mind and weak body by living outside the needs of the modern world—the demands that bills be paid, vehicles be serviced, and appointments be made and kept. Little is expected of me, and I start to rely on my wife to take charge of our family's daily life. Time and space remain curiously constricted around me unless I am outside, but being detached from the business of living is helping me heal, helping me manage my weaknesses, boosting my belief that in time, I will recover.

* ★ ★ ★ ★

My long-time friend Bob frequently drives me to Calgary for my twice-monthly check-ups. I am grateful for the opportunity to nap along the way, preparing for the battery of tests that occur on several floors of the cancer centre. I trundle along between appointments, usually exhausted by the time I meet with Dr. Stewart, my regular physician in the outpatient clinic. He is pleased with my progress despite my low level of neutrophils and liver GVHD; knowing my penchant for data, he always provides me with copies of my results. While I am no longer afraid of living, his calm and confident demeanor instills a confidence in me beyond the small medical steps I am making toward recovery.

I am also enamored with the smiles and compliments of the staff during each of my visits. It is good to feel special.

I often bring treats to the clinic and Unit 57. When I ask the receptionist if they might prefer a basket of tea, cheese, and crackers rather than the cakes, tarts, and flans I usually bring, my question is met with several resounding shouts of "No!" And when I apologize for forgetting to bring along plastic forks, I am told not to worry; no one minds licking their fingers.

The leaves of the ash trees in the backyard start to turn gold, and I watch for more signs of fall. White-crowned sparrows in the garden indicate migration is underway, and the robins disappear soon after. A few weeks later, when the juncos arrive, snow is usually soon to follow.

Bob insists we go duck hunting. He leaves me by the edge of a pond while he drives to the other side to scare birds in my direction. No matter how hard I try, I cannot get into my chest waders. I am too weak to balance on one leg, and I quickly tire of wrestling with the shapeless boots while I sit on the ground. Astonished by my weakness and growing nausea, I lie on the coarse salt grass, watching the ducks fly overhead, my gun too heavy to lift skyward.

When Bob returns, he finds me asleep in a dry bed of cattails. I tell him I did not see the ducks he flushed directly over my head. He doesn't believe me. He knows I would have shot had I been strong enough to crouch and hide in the weeds. He knows I need to go home.

Bob invites me to go deer hunting with his folks, long-time outfitters whom I first met years ago on a stormy day high in the mountains. I have enjoyed going along many times, always eager to hear their stories of guiding clients in search of elk and bighorn sheep, and their tales of encounters with grizzly bears and cougars. I know they will gladly take care of me, finding prime places where I can make a stand, but I decide the trip must wait until next year.

★ ★ ★ ★ ★

Early in the new year, I sign up for Tapestry, a five-day retreat designed for cancer patients to explore a variety of post-treatment therapies. I want to push myself harder toward recovery, and attending the workshop means I won't be shambling around the house.

The three-hour drive to the retreat location is daunting, but I have been driving carefully the past few months and am anxious to rebuild my skills behind the wheel (always my primary measure of getting well). I go slowly, staying overnight with Bob's parents half-way. I choose a bunk in the basement so I can enjoy the warmth of their wood stove.

The retreat is a wonderful opportunity to connect with others struggling to recover. Besides the typical issues of fatigue and lack of appetite, many of the participants complain about post-treatment loss of memory and reading skills, and the ability to drive, think clearly, and solve problems. There is only conjecture about how fuzzy thinking might be improved. One person suggests playing games like Solitaire on the computer to improve mental strength and capacity.

The trip is my first achievement of any kind in months. I am eager to discuss all the wonderful activities of the week with my wife, especially the value of talking about dying so you can then get on with living. Now that we can finally look ahead, I should be able to ban any worries of my death that might still be holding her back. I say we must take our daughters to Disneyland as soon as I can travel, and, secretly, I start looking at new houses.

The one-year anniversary of my transplant is two weeks away. I am excited to organize a celebration and build a guest list. There is no enthusiasm on her part, and I am left to plan a party alone, hurt and confused.

A few days later, we are sitting in the car together where I have been waiting while she has been shopping. When she returns, I mention she seems unhappy.

She announces, without forewarning, "I'm leaving."

I am too stunned to even ask why, and when we return home, I am so crushed by the happy looks on our daughters' faces that I must reach for the railing to keep myself from falling.

We remain together at home for another two months. Counseling is not an option for her: her time is spent looking for an apartment and disappearing each evening to walk the neighborhood, as she has done for months.

The girls ask, *"Why?"* and *"What about Christmas?"* We are left behind without answers, my heart splitting, and I worry how my daughters will cope with the ugly news. I hide my tears.

I have been strictly prohibited to be around animals because of my impaired immune system, but I believe a pet will help the girls cope with their fears. At my visit to the Centre the following week, I plead with staff to allow us to have a cat.

Seeing the look of anguish on my face when I tell them the reason, they finally relent, but the cat must stay indoors.

We rescue Lizzie from the animal shelter a few days later. As for me, I must find a way to rescue myself.

PART III
DRY GROUND

A lifetime of experience shapes us to meet or be crushed by such challenges as a bad divorce, the shattering of a career, a terrible illness or accident . . .

–Laurence Gonzales, *Deep Survival: Who Lives, Who Dies, and Why*

Chapter 15
Running to Nature

Wilderness is not a luxury but a necessity of the human spirit, and as vital to our lives as water and good bread.

–Edward Abbey, *Desert Solitaire*

Victoria Day, the late May long weekend that is the traditional start of camping season in Alberta. Despite being advised to stay indoors (it has only been a week since I was released from the hospital after a severe bout of shingles—a virus my doctors worry may be a prelude to further issues with my immune system), I decide to head for the foothills with my young daughters, Katie and Amy (now thirteen and eleven). We have not been camping for so long, and a few days in the wilds should help distract them from the pain and disbelief of their mother's recent departure from home. I also need a refuge to escape the doubts and fears hard on my heels.

Instinctively I choose the place where I had lived in the bush thirty years earlier while studying the habits of spruce grouse and ptarmigan (a mountain grouse that turns completely white in winter). There, I climbed mountains, crossed paths with grizzlies, and sipped the soothing elixir of alpine streams. My hair and beard grew unruly, neither cut for over two years. Beneath my Trapper Nelson, a pack board I used to carry my gear into the bush, I wore my dad's old flannel shirts. My parents called me Grizzly Adams.

Working alone season after season, miles from help, I was living my dream of being a mountain man. My idol? Jeremiah Johnson (portrayed in a movie of that name by Robert Redford).

It was a time I felt indestructible.

Immortal.

Impervious to danger.

For the trip with my girls, I have made an extensive checklist of food and gear, preparing for the inevitable extremes of spring weather in the mountains. Water jugs, cots, sleeping bags, tent, meals to cook over a wood fire, and special treats to eat while listening to ghost stories around the campfire. Because I have worn myself out gathering our supplies and equipment, the girls do most of the loading after school while I supervise. We hurry to finish packing, anxious to arrive at the campground before dark. It is twilight when we choose our site along the high banks of the Sheep River.

We are alone and I can see the girls are uneasy in the growing darkness, so I light the lantern, and we make a fire to fight the sharp cold of the night air. We make hot chocolate, and soon we are talking of adventure in the days ahead.

Where is the tent? I repeatedly search the vehicle (which is now empty except for a tarp) and the girls carefully look over the stack of gear with flashlights. There is no tent—the most essential item did not get packed. How many times had I prepared for camping without missing an item, relying solely on a mental checklist? That was, of course, before my brain was jolted awry by treatment.

I stare at the dark ground, struck with disbelief and the racing fear of failure. I have not been up so late since my sleepless nights in the hospital. I am exhausted from the strain and efforts of the day. Perhaps we should cram ourselves into the truck for the night and go home tomorrow. That would be an ugly ride home.

We do have that massive blue tarp to cover the tent in case of snow. The girls suggest we use it to make a tent, and we start to search for rope to tie between trees.

I find several feet of nylon cord. Katie and Amy remove the tie strings from their sleeping bags, but we can't tie the makeshift rope high enough to raise the heavy tarp.

The pines do not have branches to climb, but if Katie stands on my shoulders, could she tie the rope high enough to lift the tarp off the ground? No, but perhaps if I stand first on the picnic table.

Katie is tiny, but her weight almost topples me as she scrambles onto my shoulders. I fear my legs will collapse, tumbling her to the frozen ground, so I hug the tree with one arm, the coarse bark digging into my face, while gripping her slender leg with my other hand. I shake like a poplar leaf buffeted by the wind.

Katie must climb down several times before the rope is securely tied on both trees. Using branches we find in the deadfall, we fork the tarp up and over. Relieved, we laugh or cry. I do both at the same time—a newly acquired skill.

We put our cots inside the shelter and prop up the sides of our makeshift tent with sticks. I close the far end so the girls will feel safe. I place my bed sideways to block the open end from ghosts and bears. I make a show of laying the ax nearby. Tonight, I am not a cancer survivor; I am the proud father of two wonderful girls and my only concern is their happiness and safety.

Outside by the glowing campfire, I watch their shadows moving inside the tent, large in the light of the lantern. They talk excitedly while setting up their cots and arranging their stuff. They are happy, and I am somehow back in the wilderness.

When they ask to roast marshmallows before bed, I blame smoke for the tears in my eyes.

Snowy weather chases us from the area, but what a camp it has been. We took turns sleeping under the stars, jealous of the opportunity to guard the entrance to the best pup tent ever made. We collected pinecones, skipped rocks across the river, stood under a waterfall, took nature walks.

We smelled like smoke.

Basking in the warm sun held my fatigue at bay, and as I rested, I recalled the joys of past days here in the field. And as I dozed in the early morning while the girls slept, I thought of life awakening in the distant mountains and reached for the notebook under my cot:

SUNRISE CAMP

At dawn I awake to chickadees in joyful flight,
the air of spring a great delight.

Daughters yet asleep do not feel the sun,
while I think about our days of fun.

Spring winds tumble clouds on mountains near,
where the first alpine flowers above the snow are clear.

Clawed tracks the melting snow will briefly hold,
strides of a grizzly deep and bold.

Alpine ptarmigan from rocky outposts scream,
Power and life to all sweet dreams.

Displaced early from the hills, the girls want to shop before returning home. It is the first time I have ventured inside a mall since my final release from the hospital. When the girls race to the nearest store, I sit nervously on a bench, my senses overloaded with noise and neon, my vision further disoriented by the artificial light. I regret not wearing a cloth mask over my mouth to ward off the germs of the people bustling around me.

I want to go to the shelter of the truck, but the girls want me to join them on the escalator. I hold steady to the rubber handrail, more worried about the step off to the second floor than they had been as young children.

While they again disappear into the crowd, I stand alone, overwhelmed by the garish setting and unnatural environment of glass and glitz. It is a holiday, and shoppers brush around me, jostling in both directions, swinging bags and boxes. As I look for a safe spot away from the mayhem, I notice an image on an easel in the distance.

An art gallery will surely be quiet *and* safe.

As I walk closer to the painting, I gradually see it is a tiger, caught in mid-stride, staring off to the side, seeking to capture a nuance seen or heard in the darkening forest. Flecks of snow ride its fur. It is prime time to hunt elk and deer in the taiga.

The tiger and I search the misty woods together, and in those hypnotic moments, I see a forest of birch and pine— my deer stand in the Northwoods. Shadows fill the trees, and, momentarily, the snow beneath them becomes brighter. Pellets of snow are falling, turning into beads of moisture as they land on my red woolen pants and cotton gloves.

The dry brown leaves that linger on the oak brush twirl soundlessly.

I do not want to move. I know the deer will soon leave the thick bush where they have spent the day—alert to movement in the trees, the rustle of footsteps, a broken twig, a shift in the breeze. The hunters scattered throughout the woods are also watching and waiting.

Amy tugs on my arm. She says, "Dad, we need to go. It is snowing hard." Before I turn to leave, I see a nameplate attached to the frame: "Twilight - Siberian Tiger" by Robert Bateman.

The snow is steady on the way home. Big flakes, horizontal in the headlights, drift around the buildings in the small towns we pass. The girls sleep; I drive slowly on the slick roads, thinking of tigers in the snow.

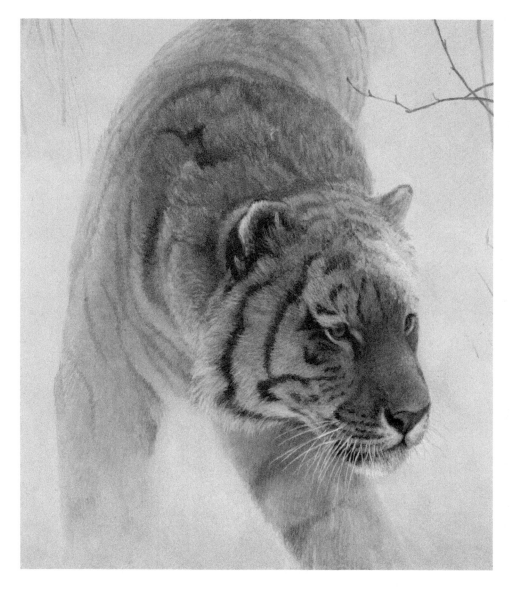

Twilight — Siberian Tiger

Chapter 16
Twilight Tiger

Look deep into nature, and you will understand everything better.

−Albert Einstein

The peace and calm that I cherished while camping soon vanish with the fears of divorce, and I have groceries to buy, lunches to make, meals to plan, laundry to do, mail to open. If only I could live in the mountains forever.

Yet the moments by the gallery do persist; I had been in awe of the tiger's beauty and strength, subconsciously entering its life, and place, in the forest. My dormant senses had come alive, and my mind was free from struggling for control. Somehow, I had also felt a touch of affection.

I have never seen a tiger in the wild—in the snow or otherwise—but I have seen a cougar in the snow.

★ ★ ★ ★ ★

It was a day many years ago, when I was in the Rockies, searching for a reputed elk trail up Green Mountain.

I was weaving through a trackless forest of dog-hair pine after a fresh snow. Feeling I was being followed, I stopped and looked back, pulling the hood off my head. There was no sound, only the hush of light snow sifting through the dull air. I peered into the black and white thicket behind me, but there was nothing to see in the maze of dense trees. My back trail was the only sign of anything moving in the silent forest.

An hour later, I began retracing my route back to the road. A new trail through unbroken snow suddenly appeared, veering away to the northwest. Cat paws, larger than my hand. Many were stride for stride over my old footprints.

I had been followed in the woods.

The prints were as clear and crisp in the powdery snow as if the animal had just stood there: the cat could only be steps ahead. I had never seen a cougar—could I see this one by following its tracks?

I twisted sideways, hunching my shoulders to slide less noisily through the spindly snow-covered branches. The ragged sound they made dragging against my coat still raced ahead of me. I strained to look past the tracks.

When the trail continued across a small clearing of stumps and slash, I stopped and brushed snow off a log. The day was almost gone, but I sat anyway in the windless twilight, my body heat filling the air pockets in my clothes, my breath rising in the still air.

I watched.

I waited.

I was getting cold.

A good moon, three quarters and waxing full, crested the ridge above me. And then something moved near the skyline. I raised my binoculars.

A cougar. Head down, calm, its stare holding me still for several heartbeats.

Stars were out.

I hiked back to the road by the white light of the moon, no longer feeling chilled.

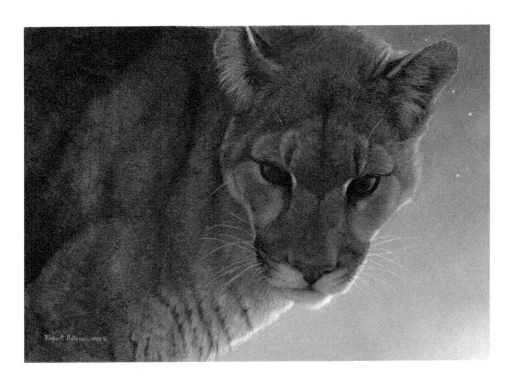

Starlight – Cougar

★ ★ ★ ★ ★

I decide to place a deposit on "Twilight."

I enter the store for the first time several days later. Wolves, eagles, bears, and lions surround me, and when I turn a corner, I am startled by a new Siberian tiger, this one hidden among snowy boughs of spruce.

Looking for my tiger, I am tense with anticipation. When I find it, I feel mist on my face, the quiet of fog. I am captured by the gaze of the tiger yet acutely alert. No other painting on display in the gallery grips me so powerfully.

Out in the bright spring sunlight, I carry the painting carefully across the parking lot, feeling invigorated by the first warm day of the year. In the poplar trees above my truck, tiny leaves are uncurling from hundreds of sticky buds; thin shadows from the branches meander across the ground. Green blades are emerging from the bleached grass.

I hear bees, and when I look up, the dread of cancer disappears. Perhaps it is the weather, or how paintings of wildlife have stimulated my spirit, or the companionship of my new friends at the gallery, but I just *know*, for the first time since those nights of fevers on Unit 57, I will make it.

★ ★ ★ ★ ★

When I return home, I place the tiger over my bed. I stand beside it, feeling the tiger's strength, anticipating its movement. When I look more intently, I can feel a tangible *energy* radiating from its muscular, yet fluid, body.

Perhaps what I am feeling is simply my imagination, like how you trick your mind into seeing the hidden images in those quirky pictures once popular in storefronts. But I recall experiencing the same powerful feelings during my days in the field, often in response to the beauty of plants and animals. I had never truly contemplated the source of that energy, but it had been real and had always rejuvenated my body and spirit.

I need to see more wildlife art; I have been deprived of nature by all the months of enforced confinement and my fear of the outdoors. I eagerly boot up the computer for the first time in months, looking for a website of art by Robert Bateman.

His paintings of animals and nature hold my focus without conscious effort and quickly become a buffer against the recurrence of depression. Eagles, colorful birds, and wolves attract my attention, but images of wild cats, especially those of solitary animals, intrigue me (when I splash water on my face and rub it around with my hands, I realize I wash my face like a cat).

I find cougars and lynx. A bobcat. An ocelot. A snow leopard, an endangered animal trying to make a living in the most spectacular mountains of my daydreams.

As I study the leopard on the screen, I imagine climbing high into the winter, surrounded by snow-packed valleys, searching for the tracks of this secretive animal, wary of avalanche, snow blindness and yeti.

I reach the top of a fog-shrouded ravine, my hair damp, my face wet. I stop to tie my boot, and when I look up, the leopard in "Out of the White" is there, beside me, caught by my unexpected appearance, its green eyes fixed onto mine. I look down, trying to seem oblivious to the encounter, the tawny-gray fur, black spots and huge paws only feet away, the thick tail trailing into the distance. I am afraid to move.

A timeless stillness captures my body and mind, eliminating the vibrations in me, and I feel again the resurgence of my awakening spirit.

The painting reminds me of *The Snow Leopard,* a book by Peter Matthiessen that has been my companion for over two decades both at home and in the field. I love the radiant prose that describes the Himalayan wilderness and the overpowering beauty of the winter landscape, but it is his quest to find himself while traveling the trails of tough nature that now has the book in my hand. I am not yet able to read long passages, but there is no need; I can readily flip to the dog-eared pages with check marks and notes in the margin.

The lessons I had learned then remain intact:

Seek the moment in a conscious way; pay attention to the present.

Quiet the mind and *feel* the rhythm of life without the hindrances of the past and uncertainties of the future.

Harness the healing power of nature.

The years of watching and waiting, the transplant, and the many months of tests and medications had always focused on keeping my body alive, defeating cancer, and coping with the damaging side effects of chemotherapy and radiation. Now I have a means to mend my soul. Each night, I go to bed with the anticipation of tomorrow, and liken myself to the wide-eyed child I once was on the night before Christmas.

I am riding high, thinking I have never felt this good before, finally free from the worries imposed by my diagnosis all those years ago.

Perhaps I could not expect the experience—like most euphoria—to last.

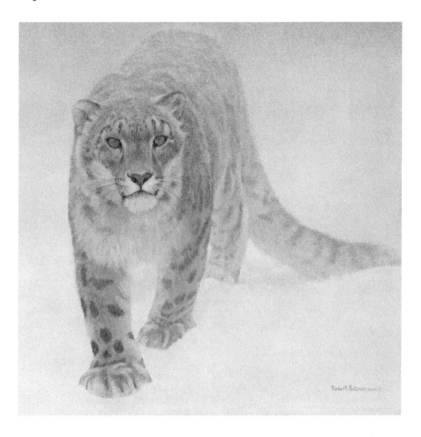

Out of the White - Snow Leopard

Chapter 17
Deer in the Headlights

Mental fatigue diminishes our ability to ignore irrelevant information, magnifies the unimportant, and makes us absolutely more prone to distraction.

–Eva M. Selhub and Alan C. Logan, *Your Brain on Nature*

Whatever is going on in my brain intensifies, and I start to see too much. Outside, I stop walking to trace a crack in the sidewalk, noting its depth and direction as it meanders through the concrete. I see a furrow in the bark on a tree and cannot walk past. I notice the sheen of stop signs at street corners, studying the fine borders between the pimpled white letters and their red background; I do not, however, see the drivers waiting for me to cross.

In the kitchen, I feel compelled to examine a mark on the floor rather than continue walking to the closet for a broom. The exponential growth in my level of perception is overwhelming—I can barely look away from crumbs by the stove, and when I do, I see fingerprints on the cupboards.

I am so distracted by minutiae that when I go to get a cup from the drying rack, I unconsciously reach for the teabags on the counter. When I head for the cupboard to get a plate, I open the refrigerator instead.

I cannot think of one thing and do another. I stop washing a dish if I listen to a random thought or look at a bowl of apples on the counter. I touch pots boiling on the stove although I know they are hot.

In the bathroom, I have considerable trouble adjusting the water temperature for a shower, alternately burning and freezing my hand several times beneath the faucet; scrolling the toilet paper roll while sitting on the can provides either too much or too little paper for the job at hand.

I wander about with a distorted sense of time and distance, as if I am stuck in dense fog. I debate when to brush my teeth; moments later when I grab my toothbrush, I see it is already wet from use.

Tomorrow, during my appointment at the outpatient clinic, I must talk to them about this: so many things are unclear.

I have never been lost in the woods, but I am lost at home.

★   ★   ★   ★   ★

Now, where are the damn urinals?

Last time I was in here, they were parked on the side wall across from the toilet stalls. They have always been there. Has the place been renovated? I spin around, becoming dizzy. I open the stalls. Just toilets. Where are they?

I walk out into the small alcove between the bathroom doors. A stylized human symbol is on the door a few feet from my face. I inspect it for several seconds and convince myself it is a male figure. Turning around, I see the indentation of a woman on the door I just came out of.

What the hell?! Have I been in the women's can?

Pushing hesitantly through the door with the manly figure, I am relieved to find there are, indeed, urinals awaiting me this time. Did anyone notice me entering or leaving the ladies' room?

Hustling to the outpatient clinic, I rationalize my mistake. I was in a rush: anyone in a hurry could have done the same thing. Now, however, I realize I have been struggling to recognize the gender symbols on washroom doors for months.

At first, I joked about how I was compensating for having a woman's bone marrow cells in me. Now, it's not so funny: I realize I have been unable to trust my instincts to recognize many formerly unmistakable designs, patterns and signs (many of them while driving).

My reception at the outpatient clinic is warm and enthusiastic; comments are always made about how well I look, whether warranted or not. I take a seat in my assigned cubicle and await the basic physical assessment that is the routine start of my twice-monthly visits. I will probably be reminded I need to start redoing all my immunizations because I have yet to schedule them at the health unit in Lethbridge.

My blood tests are comparable to those of my recent visits. I would be happy for improvements in my liver function (compromised by prolonged GVHD) and immune response (I have a low level of infection-fighting neutrophils), but these are minor problems. Physically I feel the same—always tired, insomnia, no appetite, a few bouts of incontinence, post-neuralgic symptoms from the shingles and a bunch of minor ailments (like my split thumb nails). Not altogether different from a lengthy summer stay in the field—achy muscles, mildly dazed from a lack of sleep, cravings for fruits and greens, a touch of constipation, sunburn, some bug bites (I don't like to use repellent), a few scratches, and a bruise or two, ailments fodder for hardiness. So I am confident in my physical recovery, believing I will improve with time and patience.

I skip the bathroom episode and downplay my mental lapses at home because I want to stress something else: my basic hard skills—reading, writing, and arithmetic, always the strengths I have taken for granted—have disappeared, no matter how hard I try to kick-start them.

Reading overpowers my concentration. My favorite test in grade school was reading comprehension, the timed versions on which I typically received perfect scores. Now the words flow, but lack meaning, and when I try rereading, I start to examine the font. I always prefer the pictures on a page, like a pre-schooler learning to read.

Stringing words together in a sentence while writing is a difficult task. When I try to sign my name, my hand is frozen after the initial flourish.

Simple math eludes me. When I try to add a small string of double-digit numbers in my head, I question whether the total is correct. Even counting pocket change or tabulating short columns of small numbers with a calculator challenges me. I stop trying to use recipes: I confuse units of measurement and the proper sequence of adding ingredients.

432-6583. My parents' home telephone number; the one I had to memorize, like all children starting kindergarten; the number to be given to adults if I got lost. Those seven digits have always been an indelible sequence in my mind; I have dialed them automatically countless times over decades, whether near or far from home.

Yet now this series of numbers escapes me completely. When I pick up the phone to call my folks, my hand stops short of the keypad, my index finger poised in the air awaiting instructions to tap the first digit. Previously, the numbers would have reached out to me, so automatic was the exchange between thought and action. Now the pause is permanent, the dial tone soon ringing busy in my hand. Even after being told the number, I can go no further than the four and three. When I write the number down, I fail to recognize it any more than a phone number randomly selected from the phone book.

How could I be losing such basic skills that surely have been embedded in my brain?

My nurse says I am suffering from "chemo brain" or "chemo fog." She tells me the situation is only temporary and adds the "Don't worry, we did that to you" maxim to reassure me (I learn later the technical term is cancer-treatment-associated cognitive change, and I'm angry to read that some oncologists believe it is only an *imaginary* phenomenon).

I am relieved there is a cause for my mental missteps but disturbed by the new uncertainty I now face. I knew chemotherapy would damage my body: I did not anticipate any problems in my thinking because of treatment, and I am certain I did not read or hear about any mental side effects during the years I was watching and waiting. I expected my inner voice to function as steadily and smartly as it always did to solve problems and make decisions, and to operate most efficiently during times of crisis, health-related or otherwise, as it had in the past.

My nurse suggests computer games might help rejuvenate my agitated brain pathways. When I try this at home, though, after only a few minutes of tracking cards and symbols across the screen, my mind is overwhelmed by the effort. Likewise, I only see each move as its own entity, and the repetitive thinking required to play the games soon exhausts me. Plus, the cards have numbers; my attention is drawn instead to their colors and designs.

In the weeks and months ahead, numbers continue to haunt me, and anything that needs an amount, a quantity, or a value to be gathered, counted, or measured, is met with a puzzling void.

When I try to make coffee, I am bewildered, drilled to the floor, frozen like a deer fixed by headlights. I always short out during the measurement phase. After spooning a few tablespoons of coffee into the basket, I lose count of the number of scoops. Is that five or six scoops? Wait, perhaps it is only four? The debate inside my head only leads to further indecision.

Standing at the kitchen counter, full spoon in hand, suspended in midair, I am not sure what to do next. My psychomotor skills, depending on near-simultaneous brain and motor activity, are paralyzed, freezing me in place.

Why does a deer freeze when hit by bright light? The sudden flash creates temporary blindness, and rather than flee into danger, the animal stands still until its eyes, equipped with exceptional night vision, readjust to the dazzling brightness.

Shocked by the chemo, I too am "flash-blind." Some of the chemotherapy drugs I received traveled to my brain, attacking nerve cells, altering my neural pathways. Signals do not arc cleanly between my synapses, impeding transmission, causing neurons to bounce into oblivion rather than reach their proper destinations. My thoughts often come in starbursts that race away into a haze before I can grasp them. And the forces of chemo brain now threaten to rob me of the soothing effects of wildlife art.

I go outside to escape the unrelenting chaos that controls my mind. I hear the shrill blast of a blue jay, a bird that is calling again now that fall has arrived. The crazy laughter of a flicker, another loud bird quiet during the summer, resounds in the neighborhood.

I yearn to be surrounded by wild nature.

Chapter 18
Against the Wind

In a single leaf falling on a windless day, time folded
its long stretch into a moment and slipped past
right before my eyes.

> – Sooyong Park and John Valiant,
> *Great Soul of Siberia: Passion, Obsession, and One Man's*
> *Quest for the World's Most Elusive Tiger*

It is October, and I am in Wisconsin because my mother is
severely ill with cancer. I have gladly deflected my family's
concerns about my recovery, shifting the conversations instead
toward my mom's failure to respond to her treatment for bone
cancer. Together, she and I sit quietly, holding hands. It is the
last time we will see each other.

My friend since childhood invites me to float a river while
I am in Green Bay. Bill and I began school together in kindergarten. He calls me "Fess," a nickname he applied while we
were in high school. Nature and conservation bond our friendship even when our time together occurs years apart. We will
be paddling through the splendid fall colors of the hardwood
forest that bounds the nearby Plover River.

The river is shallow in autumn and flows gently through the
countryside. Bill has been down the river many times, and with
him guiding us from the stern, I am not worried about being

on my first canoe trip since the transplant. He has insisted I must relax in the bow, helping paddle only to avoid sandbars and fallen trees along the shoreline. There are no rapids.

Bill has always had my back, ever since we were atop the mountains of snow plowed from our grade school playground, standing back-to-back as we hurled chunks of snow at the attackers below us, unbeatable as we played king of the hill. He blames me for all the mischief we have made over the years, but I remind him he was most often the leader of the wild "stampedes" that ran through the basement of our grade school.

There is little breeze and full sun as we push off from the bank. The bow swings downstream and I feel the solid tug of the current; I have forgotten how being on water grasps my being. The musty scent of wet, decaying leaves infuses the air.

"Oh my God," I exclaim, feeling myself moving effortlessly without the usual crushing drain of energy that occurs with anything I do. Floating is freedom: I trail my hands in the water, amazed at the maple leaves that spin and sail alongside me. I marvel at their different colors and sizes, some perfectly shaped, others frayed along the edges and pocked with holes. I pluck some of the red ones, my favorites, as they spin through the eddies and back to me. The water is richly colored with tannin, very cold, and icy to the taste. I am so enthralled that I forget to paddle. Bill does not mind, steering us easily downstream.

I spot some red berries on the opposite shore and make Bill cross the river to investigate and identify. High-bush cranberries, shrunken by frost. I taste them: very tart and seedy. They will be high-quality food for winter birds. Paddling back to the other side, we cross shallow water, maybe two feet deep. Here smooth pebbles shine along the sandy riverbed.

Bill holds our position in the current and shifts his weight while I roll up my sleeve, leaning over the side to scoop a handful of the gem-like stones. As the best of the shiny pebbles go into my pocket, a kingfisher rattles across the river. The bird is a male, and we wonder, if pools of minnows remain open after freeze-up, how long he will stay during the winter.

Ahead, cedars block the shore, green needles touching the water. Bill says wood ducks—an eastern species that I have not seen in many years—often hide beneath the low-hanging limbs. The drakes have multicolored iridescent plumage—green, black, purple, blue—a crest, a red eye, a white stripe, patches of reddish brown and buffy gold feathers. What if we saw one?

We are floating within feet of the branches when I see a swatch of brownish, grayish-blue feathers moving ahead on some rocks above the water. Only when I see the white trim around the eye and the wispy crest do I recognize the bird—a female wood duck. I barely see the ornate male before they rocket downstream, low on the water and out of sight around the next bend.

I happily recite how wildlife biologists saved wood ducks from extinction by preserving crucial habitat and enlisting the public to build and place nest boxes in swampy areas. Bill knows the story, but acts like he is hearing it for the first time.

Farther downstream, crows make a racket. Some perch on the leafless limbs of an oak, throwing their heads back. Others dart back and forth at an overhang of cedar branches. We watch, but whatever creature has attracted the crows is hidden beneath the thick boughs. Finally, a great horned owl breaks from the cover. The ruckus continues downstream: we hope the owl quickly finds refuge from his pursuers.

An hour on the river and at each new bend, nature pulls me further into its embrace. For the first time in years, I pinch myself to make sure what I see and feel is real. I eventually notice the wind funneling upstream, pulling dry leaves from the hardwoods and swirling them upriver. The spindly tops of the big cedars, caught in the leading edge of the storm, start to sway.

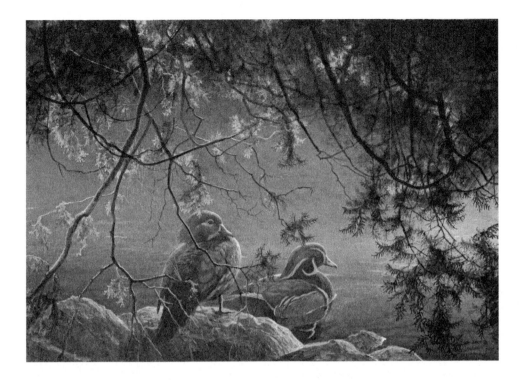

On the Pond - Wood Ducks

Soon we are trapped in a shallow, open, marshy part of the river, fully exposed to a fierce headwind that overpowers the slow current that was helping us downstream. We are glued to the river surface; my hands are trembling and I can barely lift my arms. Bill is tiring in the stern, just able to keep the bow forward. The sun strains weakly through the advance of gray-white tumbling clouds.

I have said nothing to Bill about my ever-present fatigue, but now that we are stuck in the middle of the river and I am helpless, I shout at him from the bow:

"I'm not a cripple, you know!"

But I'm angry at myself and my feeble efforts to help him paddle against the wind.

Each new gust whips the cattails lining the shore, shredding the cigar-shaped heads, tossing fluff into the sky that sticks to our coats. I know I can't wade through those thick reeds to reach dry ground.

Rain is imminent; we can smell it.

As we retreat upstream, Bill sees a narrow side channel into the cattails. He jumps into the water and pushes us to safety while I sit, helplessly exhausted, in the bow. He lands the canoe in the shelter of an oxbow surrounded by trees. I climb the low bank, thankful to lie down on a patch of green grass.

There are some big oak trees overhead; they look like the ones that still live in the yard behind my parents' home. Unable to join hands as we spread our arms around their trunks, we marvel at the trees' girth. They remind us of the "Good Oak" essay in *The Sand County Almanac* written by Aldo Leopold, a tribute to the age and longevity of such mighty specimens. We wonder if passenger pigeons, extinct for over a hundred years (one of the last wild birds was shot in Wisconsin), might have found food or shelter in the branches above us.

It is a short walk across the pasture to the nearest road, where we can hitch a ride to our car. Bill can come back to retrieve the canoe after the storm.

Reflecting on the aborted trip that night as I lie beneath the old deer head in my childhood bedroom, I know it will join the lore of our many previous adventures, but I am depressed, and totally disgusted by my lack of strength and endurance. I have always enjoyed thunderstorms, blizzards, the challenges of stormy weather—harsh nature that has made me feel the strength and energy of life. My motto of "tough nature brings out the best in a man" seems like it now applies to a previous life.

Will I ever get back to where I was before cancer? Is that not the goal of recovery? If the fatigue I am carrying like the plague does not abate, I will never hike again in the mountains, never reach the high alpine where the peaks touch the heavens. Never see a jungle trail, never pick my way through a marsh.

Never be calm.

Chapter 19
A New Body

Where I had once run easily along the bicycle paths
beside the Bow River, I was now lucky just to walk.
If I tried to jog, I became exhausted very quickly.
It was a constant battle not to become demoral-
ized and lament that what I had lost, rather than
celebrate that which I still had.

–Alan Hobson, *Climb Back from Cancer*

My bone marrow transplant has been declared a success. I have
made sure of that by demanding extra bone marrow biopsies.
This time, after Dr. Stewart insists my blood tests are accurate
and reliable evidence of remission, I tell him the field biologist
in me needs the data and will endure the pain for the extra
proof. I persist until he tells me to turn and face the wall.

After touching my back in several spots, searching for a clear
place to punch the needle, he says to his intern, with a hint
of disbelief, "Look at all these scars. You can sure tell a long-
term survivor."

I consider the scars measures of toughness.

After the procedure, I hesitate to share my final concern of
the day—the one that is never on the lists of questions I fax Dr.

Stewart each day before my appointments. It seems ungrateful after surviving cancer-free for four years.

I explain that my weeks and months are slipping aimlessly by as every morning I awake dog-ass tired. Despite getting consistent good news from him from every source: biopsies, bloodwork, chest x-rays, ultrasounds, eye exams, dental visits and lung function tests, I live solely under a heavy lid of fatigue that never lifts.

Because every day is a dismal repeat of the day before, I say I feel like Bill Murray's character in the movie *Groundhog Day*, the weatherman who finds himself caught in a time loop, reliving February 2nd again and again. Like that character, every attempt I make to rebuild myself ends in failure. When I climb the basement steps and feel invigorated by the effort, I add steps to my routine the following day. Sometimes, I feel strengthened by the extra work; other times I get bounced onto the couch for the afternoon. Other times, walking a half-mile feels like an ideal amount of exercise: the next time, the same distance turns the effort of preparing a simple dinner into a marathon.

My frustration extends to the everyday chores of living in what I term the "modern world." Before I became ill, if tasks around the house began to pile up, I would catch up by working evenings and a Saturday or Sunday. Now, pushing hard backfires or is counterproductive, adding to the strains of chemo brain and increasing my vulnerability to depression. I have no energy to go outside.

My wish is for just a single day when I can feel the same as I did before I got cancer—just one day when I awake, roll over, pivot, and put my feet on the floor, feeling refreshed, ready to do whatever I want, for however long I wish. Just one of the old days when I could work in the field and come back home without worrying how I would feel the next day. Now the scant energy I have is quickly depleted by the simple tasks of daily living and never restored by rest, sleep or exercise. I am trapped in an unreliably weak body, one that is merely a brittle shell of its former self.

My tears are flowing as I explain all this to Dr. Stewart.

"Perhaps you would like to meet Dr. Hicks," he suggests.

★ ★ ★ ★ ★

Dr. Heather Hicks works specifically with survivors of breast cancer, a group plagued with serious long-term fatigue. In my first appointment with her, I tell her I'm constantly tired and poleaxed by low energy, wandering about half-awake, feeling stunned throughout each day. Yet my body buzzes and jangles with tension. I shake my set of keys to mimic the effect, adding that if I stand too long in front of the mirror, I quiver.

I tell her that I try to rest, but rest has been no remedy for my continuous lack of energy. "More rest," I complain, is always the advice from friends and family in response to my complaints, sometimes almost dismissively, as if I should be healthier by now.

I add that I was never so continuously exhausted while working outdoors, even after miles of wading, hiking, climbing, or paddling. My energy would return after a sound meal, a few hours of relaxation, and a single good night's sleep. I had the ability to push hard to the limits of my endurance, knowing I could always recharge and rally furiously day after day, week after week, month after month, to finish my projects. Now fearful of pushing too hard, I treat spurts of energy as warnings to stop what I am doing; too much activity means I will crash and burn, often for days thereafter.

The best I can muster is being a half-day man, a phrase used often by my dad. At 83 years of age and never having believed in healthy eating or exercise, it seems like a logical situation for him, but it isn't what I want the rest of my life.

"Are you able to exercise regularly?" she asks.

"No. I try walking, but how far I go one day is too much the next. I can only walk short distances, but sometimes the shortest loops I walk around the neighborhood seem like trails in the Rockies."

Dr. Hicks stresses that fatigue and tiredness are not the same thing. Defining fatigue as "extreme tiredness" is misleading. Being exhausted by physical exertion is being tired. Overdoing something, being drained of energy by difficult or sustained effort—that leads to tiredness. The remedy for tiredness is rest and refueling the body with proper food and drink; the cure is the healing powers of restful sleep.

Fatigue is unrelenting weariness, a physical state impervious to the factors that allow a body to recover from tiredness. It is a revealing distinction of my condition, and explains why fatigue is an unforgiving menace to my recovery from cancer. I find consolation in clarification, and in learning that fatigue also intensifies anxiety and memory loss.

What else can I say about myself? I miss the dopey feeling that signals a smooth descent into sleep. When I lie down, my mind and body vibrate with nervous energy until a hidden force slams down on my consciousness (Dr. Hicks attributes the tension to latent trauma). I wake often with the jitters, only noting by the time elapsed on the clock that I must have slept. Throughout the day, I feel heavy when I move: I would like to try swimming, but I am too weak to tread water. Outside I stumble over imaginary objects. And without nature beneath my feet, I feel wounded, crippled, more dead than alive.

Dr. Hicks asks if I have mentioned my deplorable fitness to staff at the outpatient clinic. Yes, but I've been told I need to accept my new body (I'm always told to listen to my *new* body), and that I will learn to read its signals about when to rest and sleep. But there have been no signals, so I've been advised to rest without the sense of being tired. I'm already trying to eat without ever being hungry: eating without hunger pangs brings no joy.

This new body I have doesn't know how to tell me what it wants. I am back to watching and waiting for signals, an especially discouraging task when I want to race with life after the near-miss of dying.

I add that I see and feel everything with a nearly mind-blowing intensity that drains my thoughts (except when I observe nature, which usually calms me), and when I confide that my four years of remission include losing my job of twenty-two years, divorce, and the anxiety of being a single parent to two teenage girls, I start to cry.

Dr. Hicks says I am clinically disabled by fatigue, my symptoms as deep as that of any of her other cancer patients. Fatigue is making me mentally tired, and combined with chemo brain, is likely affecting my mood. If so, I am caught in a self-reinforcing loop in which fatigue, mood, and fuzzy thinking feed off each other and keep depression in the game.

"How might a day unfold?" she asks.

"I wake up tired," I say, "my eyes scratchy and burning, and my head is cloudy. I wonder if I slept. I feel the divot in my groin, checking for pain. I hope I can stand up without getting dizzy. I might have a headache."

"What do you do next?"

"I may eat something, but usually I just have coffee. I might decide to write an e-mail to my sister asking about my dad's declining health. It takes an hour to type a short page because it takes me forever to find the letters on the keyboard. Often I hit some invisible key that erases my work. If I don't start over right away, I lose my thoughts. It's frustrating because sometimes I have to start over two or three times."

"Are you willing to do homework?" she asks. I smile at the thought that jumps to mind.

"I've always done my homework in school—and often for others too. Why, I even filled out my buddy's entire science book in grade six for Sister Pius" (that was also Bill, who was more interested in practicing his jump shot and chasing girls).

More seriously, I add, "I always do my homework; it's like research to me."

Dr. Hicks describes my task. I am to monitor my energy levels at regular intervals throughout the day over the next four weeks. I am to record the timing of my daily activities, especially naps, and the time I go to bed each night. I am to note changes in my general health as well, including my frame of mind. Finally, it is important to record my food intake, noting any changes in my typical lack of hunger and taste.

She encourages me to add any other insights I have about the nature of my condition, current and historical, personal and professional. I am pleased with her comprehensive and numerical approach to improving my health, sensing I have found a strong ally in my struggle to become a whole person.

We also share some humor and laughter about my predicament. I tell her I like old western movies.

"Is this too much work for you?" she asks as I prepare to leave.

"I was once a hound for data," I say. "I will bring you my results, and the binder full of notes I have compiled over the past decade."

"I look forward to it," she says.

When I bring in my homework at our next appointment, I am humming a well-practiced but poorly performed rendition of the theme song from the cult western *The Good, The Bad, and The Ugly*, (starring Clint Eastwood, the actor my mom's friends say I look like). I have recently watched the movie for the hundredth time, hence the idea for my uniquely nonprofessional introduction to my findings of the past month.

A Good Day: Four to five hours of passable energy so I can function normally around the home, which includes the occasional foray for groceries, car maintenance, a school or medical appointment, a walk around the neighborhood. Success here encourages me to do more, but is blunted by fatigue.

A Bad Day: Two to three hours of muted energy a day, primarily focused on household chores, including some laundry.

An Ugly Day: A handful of 15-20 minute spurts of energy dedicated to making meals while fighting the urge to lie down all day, fingers of phantom pain tracing the earlier course of shingles down my face warning me to go slowly.

I explain that guessing which of these days will fill a week or sequence of weeks is a crapshoot. A closer look at the data confirms the unpredictable nature of my energy.

Dr. Hicks tells me about an upcoming study by the University of Calgary's Faculty of Kinesiology that will examine the potential benefits of moderate aerobic exercise on the energy levels of cancer survivors. The target group is bone marrow transplant survivors, the group most critically impaired by chronic cancer-related fatigue.

The chief investigator, Dr. David Smith, is an expert at training Olympic athletes, including speed skaters and cross-country skiers. His specialty is the design of conditioning programs that help speed recovery after intense bouts of high performance physical activity.

This will be serious stuff, a yearlong commitment. There will be out-of-pocket expenses and overnight trips every month to Calgary to participate in successive days of exercise and testing. Candidates will soon be selected for participation in the study. Am I interested in applying?

Am I? I have tried to exercise, but each routine has led to energy blackouts and relapses after barely noticeable gains in my level of fitness. No activity has promised ongoing benefits, so I no longer routinely do anything that causes physical exertion.

I will never find another program with so much potential to restore my health and give me the chance to once again do fieldwork.

I carefully complete the many forms that describe my health since my transplant, concerned any errors might disqualify me from the study. There is a big section about depression—I suspect negative feelings would impair the will to train for the lengthy duration of the program. I cheat a little here, afraid of being eliminated from contention.

My interview seems to go well. Two weeks later, I become one of the twelve survivors selected from a pool of 222 candidates to start the program. I rush down the hallway to tell Dr. Hicks I have won the lottery.

★　★　★　★　★

There is a team of technicians waiting for me in the exercise laboratory when I arrive for my orientation. The setup for testing is extensive; just like a professional athlete, I am hooked up to a series of computers that will monitor my oxygen intake and heart rate as I ride a stationary bike. At regular intervals, my blood will be tested to assess the build-up of lactic acid. I am fascinated by all the data to be gathered and how they will be analyzed in the months ahead.

Dr. Smith shows me the functions of the bike, emphasizing that I am not in competition with the other participants. There is no winning or losing. The objective is to determine if my specific level of fatigue will respond to a customized routine of exercise. Everyone will have a unique program.

The technicians insist I must stop riding if I feel too weak to continue cycling, and I am told it would be foolhardy to think I must "go hard or go home" while setting a baseline to measure my future progress. Nonetheless, I know I will push myself hard, once again determined to be the best patient ever.

I begin to pedal. As it becomes more difficult, I focus on a poster in front of me depicting the symbols of the Olympic Games. The resistance increases on the bike and the overlapping rings on the poster begin to get blurry. I am asked repeatedly if I can go on, questions to which I nod my head because a mask is over my mouth.

I'm getting dizzier. But I refuse to quit. When I sense I might pass out, I hear yelling to stop, and soon several hands are clapping me on the back, applauding my effort. I feel I have accomplished something for the first time in years.

My body responds well in the weeks ahead. I regain my balance and walk with a purposeful stride rather than a wandering shuffle. As my endurance increases, my fatigue starts to abate, and I no longer hesitate to carry more than one load of laundry a day to the basement. Rather than using my disability parking pass, I stop in the outer rows of parking lots.

I begin to feel euphoric after test rides each week and those I complete in the gym back home. I feel like I am being injected with energy, developing a tough new body. The fitness data confirm my subjective feelings of gaining strength and stamina. My technicians show me the charts that portray my improvement and make me feel like an all-star.

I drive through spring blizzards to keep my tests on schedule. I even insist on going directly to the lab from the airport after being away for my mother's funeral. I have a lifeline, and a responsibility, and I cannot let go.

One year later, at the end of the study, I know how to interpret the tables and figures that describe my dramatic resurgence in fitness. I also have explicit "before and after" data: percent body fat, a decrease from 20% to 16.7%, resting heart rate, a drop from 110 beats per minute to 87, blood pressure, 140/95 down to 122/78.

But I do not need the hard evidence to know I have rejoined the land of the living. Remission from cancer meant survival, but walking and biking without fear through the city parks near home means I am alive. My daughters convince me I am ready to test my stamina with a day hike. Not just any hike, but the one at my favorite place in the mountains: the Highwood Pass.

Chapter 20

A Golden Day

I am well again, I came to life in the cool winds and
crystal waters of the mountains.

–John Muir (1838-1914), early advocate for wilderness preservation

Rising to nearly 8,000 feet, the Highwood Pass is reached by
the highest paved road in Canada. The thin air snaps sharply
at the summit, where a trail climbs steeply above the trees to a
bowl of alpine meadows surrounded by jagged peaks marked
with snow year-round.

Katie and Amy have hiked with me to the alpine several
times, even as children (and they know I hope one day they
will return to scatter a handful of my ashes across the boulders
and scree). Now they tease me that *if* I can reach the top of
the trail, I will see bighorn sheep, pikas, ravens, marmots, wild-
flowers, and maybe ptarmigan, knowing it was here that I once
fondly studied the elusive birds with my German shorthaired
pointer, Bonnie.

The birds were uncommon and secretive, easy to walk past
as they hid in piles of rocks, their mottled plumage of brown,
gray, white, and black strongly mimicking the colors and patterns of the lichen-covered boulders. Without the dog's keen
nose, I would have missed most of the birds, especially in early

winter, when they turned white. Even when they were invisible, roosting beneath the snow, Bonnie would stop until the nervous birds burst into the air, often only feet from her nose.

The day breaks beautifully, a sliver of moon hanging above the tallest peak. I follow the girls' lead and a few minutes from the trailhead, we walk into the solid, rich aroma of fir trees that reminds all of us of Christmas. I remind the girls, yet another time, that we must always be mindful of grizzly bears. Announce your presence wherever you go. Never walk through brush or along streams that would muffle the sounds of your progress. Avoid the dense patches of stunted trees at the timberline where bears could rest for the day. Note changes in the wind. Practice keeping your bear spray handy and how to use it.

We stop often for snacks and water, and twice, when we see fresh bear diggings, we pause for minutes before going ahead.

As we climb through the last of the trees, we are met by the comforting warmth of the sun on our backs, and I breathe deeply of the crystalline air. A narrow band of meltwater tumbles over nearby rocks, and I hurry to get an icy mouthful.

The hike is an ever-unfolding adventure of sights, sounds, and feelings without sensing the passage of time. Each step reveals something new. And I finally feel energy recharging relentlessly inside of me.

★   ★   ★   ★   ★

When I awake the next morning to sore muscles, I realize I have not felt quite this good in years.

Replaying the images of the day, I tearfully forge my feelings into written words. They become a tribute to Kathy, my donor. She has always called a gorgeous summer day spent outside, free from work and worry, a "golden" day.

GOLDEN DAY

Fireweed and purple aster were still in bloom,
As we started to hike from the Highwood Pass that August afternoon.
At first we climbed through spruce and subalpine fir,
A dense forest where the wind did not stir.

Switchbacks led us ever higher on this day so fair,
Soon we stopped for breath in the high Rocky Mountain air.
The trees were smaller, more twisted and broken with our ascent,
For into many storms and strong winds they have bent.

We anticipated the open sky alpine meadow and sharp peaks with glee,
A sight once familiar but one I doubted I would ever come again to see.
And, yes, above timberline we finally arrive,
The alarms of ground squirrels noting we'd come alive.

All around we saw folded towering sculpted snowy peaks,
So bold in a cobalt sky. No one speaks.
We follow the worn path through dried heath and rock scree,
Memories and the present magic of this place for us to see.

Along the trail a ptarmigan brood, hen and chicks, showed no fear,
Despite our approach ever so near.
Next a hawk-like shadow rode down the talus fast and black,
A raven falling down the trail at our back.

Ground squirrels, golden-mantled, also shared our way,
So too the marmot chipmunk and pika that in the alpine stay.
We ate our lunch in the shade of big rocks near a snow-melt stream,
While we talked and laughed excitedly, as if in a dream.

We forgot the time; it was the nature of the place,
And now it was dusk, time to go, careful of our space.
The forest was dark in shadow, evening wind blowing into our face,
But with knowledge and caution, we did not hurry our pace.

For grizzly bear diggings we had seen along the trail,
Thus blind corners we approached loudly without fail.
The trailhead was a welcome sight and the end of this joyful day,
For which we thanked the Lord for the health to pass this way.

The verse arrives unbidden. Perhaps because when I am outdoors, my emotions dominate my thinking. I feel more creative, and less analytical, less scientific than I did before treatment.

Maybe it is serendipity at play. One of my doctors once mused that he believed bone marrow transplants affected patients in ways that were not yet understood.

And seeing ptarmigan primes my desire to study wildlife again. I believe if I can just regain a little measure of my former hardiness, I can deliver a solid effort.

Chapter 21

Back to the Field

One of my passions is walking on this wonderful planet, in the wild areas where encounters with animals can always occur. The rhythm of my steps stimulated me to go farther and further. It is a kind of meditation.

–Carl Brenders, *Pride of Place – The Art of Carl Brenders*

My search for a return to the field leads to a crude gate of bent sticks and pieces of fence woven into a tangle of rusty barbed wire. A white metal sign is nailed to the cracked corner post: "Travel at Your Own Risk." The black letters are punched through with bullet holes.

I have not seen another vehicle since leaving the highway an hour ago. Only miles of gravel road and quarter-sections of pasture waiting for cattle, and grain fields waiting for seed. It is mid-March, too early for activity in the rural landscape.

It has been safe to scan the flat gray sky and idle fields for wildlife with only one eye on the road, something I used to do whenever I was behind the wheel. And I am handling the road better, my foot once again automatically switching from the gas to the brake.

I pour a cup of coffee and stretch my legs. The narrow trail ahead follows a canal that will turn muddy in light snow or rain. It will be dicey to travel even with four-wheel drive. The water, a steely streak of ice at the bottom of the ditch, will soon supply several prairie ponds and marshes where Ducks Unlimited, the premier wetland conservation organization in the country, is restoring the habitat after years of drought and drainage.

I ponder whether sliding off the dike into the silty water (and drowning) or an errant round of buckshot poses the greater risk. Either way, the proposed study area starts here, and I feel at home.

The job is to count waterfowl: ducks, geese, swans, herons, grebes, coots, and shorebirds (affectionately called "peeps" by many birders), one day a week, from spring migration until the end of August to determine which species are using which wetlands. The ponds will be fully flooded next year, so the data will be a baseline—like my first WBC counts years ago—to assess future changes in bird use and abundance. The study is to continue for several years; it is a superb opportunity to regain my professional identity as a wildlife biologist.

The last time I tried to go out in the field, before my transplant, I nearly went down for the count. However, then I was studying those flighty songbirds. Ducks can be counted on cloudy and mildly windy days, and are my favorite group of birds, and marshes are my favorite habitat. I have been fond of them both my entire life.

★   ★   ★   ★   ★

Marshes lined the dead-end road to my grandma's cottage on the shore of Lake Michigan where as a boy I spent my summers. Broken couches and busted refrigerators added to the dangers supposedly lurking in the swampy water—quicksand, water moccasins, and snapping turtles that could easily bite through the wooden handle of the net I used to catch frogs.

Frogs were so abundant in the short grass along the shoulder that they jumped en masse with almost every step. I caught them by the hundreds. The big ones became frog legs fried with butter in cast-iron pans by my mom and Aunt Shirley. This treat, sprinkled with salt and pepper, was served hot on paper plates to the kids and adults waiting eagerly outside at the picnic table.

Ducks were common, and as a little boy, I had ridden on my dad's back with a burlap sack of decoys, my small hands clutched around his neck, the black water sloshing between the cattails far below my feet. I was afraid to fall off into what he later called "loonshit."

When I was older, I clung to the rough bench of a storm-battered wooden skiff, wide awake before dawn as we bounced over the dark waves leading to the duck blind. Later in the morning, I would guard the decoys while my dad went for walks, watching the sky for tell-tale specks that might be ducks. By then I had seen many scary animals on the covers of my dad's sporting magazines. Dad never said anything about wolves or bears, but beaver, big weasels (mink) and muskrats certainly hid in the reeds. I had my BB gun—it felt safe being armed.

Ducks later got me kicked off the high school football team. My dad was out duck hunting when a big northeaster was pounding Green Bay, and the rafts of ducks that usually sat far out on the lake were barrelling into the calm water near shore. That night, Dad said the ducks had sailed heedlessly into his decoys and he was sorry I hadn't been along (most of our outings had been during "bluebird days," when we rarely saw ducks and Dad never fired a shot).

I skipped school the next two days. I was a good student, so my teachers didn't mind my absence too much, but missing practice meant the end of my football career.

I didn't mind being punted off the team. I was on the third string anyway, and as a member of the "pounders," I got hit by the starters every day in practice, sometimes so hard I got injured (my legacy: a weak ankle that often twists while hiking). At least I had warmed up prior to a game at fabled Lambeau Field, the home stadium of the Green Bay Packers, before those two unforgettable days with Dad.

★ ★ ★ ★ ★

The first pond, nestled in the rolling grassland just beyond the gate, is narrow enough to throw a stone across. The elevated height of the dike is ideal for viewing its surface, and once the ice melts, it will be a shallow pool without reeds or cattails where birds can hide. It will be easy to count ducks from the window of the truck without disturbing them.

I soon realize most of the wetlands are close to the trail; I can use a spotting scope to identify any birds too far away for binoculars. And the sparse vegetation in all the ponds will rarely block my view. There are also several hills near the road to use, if needed, as vantage points for the larger marshes.

I walk around the shores of a couple of ponds, testing my legs on the uneven ground. A rolling snow shower is coming from the foothills to the west, wispy streaks of cloud touching the ground.

I debate. I completed the reconnaissance, coffee in hand, in a leisurely two hours. There is no reason for any overnight trips since I am only two hours from home. If it is raining or too windy, I can postpone the survey for a day or two. If I am tired or sick, I can also wait a day or two. And I've driven today without worrying about causing an accident.

I can use my truck as a blind to count birds at most of the ponds, doing what I had once derided as windshield biology. But some of my colleagues, whom I teased as wimps, had collected great data sitting in their seats watching the undisturbed wildlife a short distance outside.

The study seems weatherproof and should be fatigue-proof. Even foolproof.

Bits of snow drift about and I try to catch them on my tongue. I attempt to track single flakes but too many of them land in my eyes, making me blink.

Walking in small circles, I study the broken stems and empty seed heads of the weathered grasses. Aimlessly, I kick at the bigger clumps, causing a vole to dart to a safer place. Three magpies appear in the distance.

How many birds will I need to count? I am still struggling with numbers, six years since my treatment. Will I have to relearn how to identify any of them, like I had to with my parents' phone number? There will be sixty to seventy different species.

Bigger snowflakes start falling across the silent landscape and I feel them landing on my head. The little hills are gone and snow is settling on the ground. I may be driving home in a spring blizzard.

Tears wet my face. I can do this study. And, dammit, I can do it well.

Chapter 22
Windshield Biology

A steady stream of magpies winged back and forth over my head like stunt planes on a popular flight path. The air was as crisp as pears, and a small breeze ruffled the tips of the new grass

–Susan Chernak McElroy, *Why Buffalo Dance*

Survey 1

The day is gray, winter still in the sky. Wind-driven snow sifts across the road from the nearby drifts.

The first two ponds are frozen. A narrow ring of water runs along the shoreline of the next pond and a dark string of ducks is busy along the edge of the ice. Divers.

A pair of redheads bobs to the surface. A few feet away, I see a cluster of bluebills (or lesser scaup), seven males and two females. What are the others? I have to record this. I spill my coffee as I reach for my notebook.

Hey, more birds on the far side. Smaller and diving for a longer time. Wait, wait . . . buffleheads . . . no, yeah, buffleheads, all right! How many—how many males, how many females? Count again to be sure. Get writing before you forget what you see.

Put down the coffee!

There is also another pair, but I need a closer look. I crank the spotting scope to a higher power and aim for the lead duck. Dark brown head. Gray flanks on gray water.

More power. Dark bill, a pale patch at the tip? The head, round with a bright eye. Common goldeneye, a female. Nice.

The male slides into view; a large white spot on its face, a yellow eye, white flanks. He chases her and they disappear under the water. Cool.

I examine the next closest bird. A drake bluebill, tiny beads of water standing on his black breast feathers. Then a blur of motion, a splash, a soft ripple of gray water. I imagine the chase for food at the bottom of the pond, the stark feel of the icy water. I do not want to look away.

I drive slowly along the trail, although I nearly spin the truck into the ditch when I jerk the wheel to glimpse a burly coyote racing across the prairie behind me. My progress sweeps flocks of horned larks off the gravel and I pause to avoid the tardy ones, stopping to identify the snow buntings among them. The larks are here to stay, the buntings heading north to the Arctic.

While scanning the skies for rough-legged hawks, big buteos also migrating north, I slide off the trail to the edge of a frozen pond. I am glad I have four-wheel drive.

With so little open water, no pond has many ducks. I have time to dally, and each observation is an entity I can ponder without the constraints of time I usually associate with bird counts. I examine the fine details of every species—wigeon, pintail, canvasback—absorbed by the vibrant colors, patterns and textures of plumage as if I had never seen them before, further intrigued by the behavior of individual birds.

Clouds pass before the sun creating shadows that drift across the ground. The throaty call of a raven tags along.

I easily finish the survey by mid-morning. My tally is 42 ducks, eighteen Canada geese, six swans, and three killdeer. As I look through my notes, a mountain bluebird lands on the barbed wire outside my window, a deep sky-blue that defies the plain brown of the dormant ground. The breeze rustles its feathers, briefly upsetting its balance. Where has he come from? The Baja? Texas? Oklahoma? A long journey, thousands of miles.

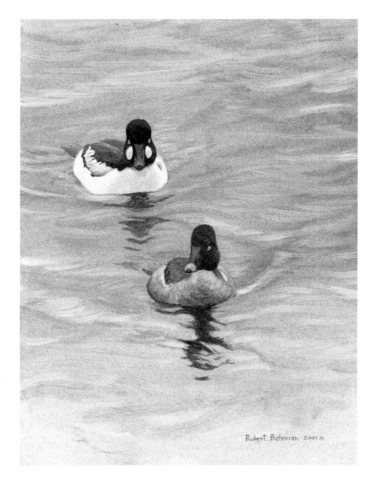

Goldeneye Pair

I close my eyes, drifting to the tune of my awakened senses, trying to etch the moment in my mind forever. When I awake with a start, the wire is bare and the bird is gone.

Seeking shortcuts on the way home, I realize the highway portion I traveled to the study area includes the section of road where I had been sick returning home from the cancer centre after radiation. Then, I could never have guessed a single turn would have led me directly to this refuge, a gentle wilderness hidden so discreetly across the miles of prairie.

That night in bed I replay the stunning memories of the day (like I did as a youth at the deer shack). Thirty years have passed since such glorious images of birds and marshes took me to sleep.

★ ★ ★ ★ ★

My grandpa loaned me $300, the cost of my first car, so I could drive to the Delta Waterfowl Research Station in southern Manitoba. I was going to be a field assistant after my third year of college.

I learned to identify every species of duck living in the marsh. Dabbling ducks. Diving ducks. Adult ducks. Male and female ducks. Flightless ducks and broods of ducks. I also trapped ducks, banded ducks, and counted ducks from canoes, airboats and float planes.

I dreamed of ducks. And I learned the names of the plants that were duck habitat.

Delta was also more than ducks. I awoke to a teeming variety of bird life that lived in the pond outside the bunkhouse windows. Soon pelicans, terns, coots, grebes, swans, geese, and an array of shorebirds—avocet, willet, dowitcher, sandpiper—warblers and blackbirds were circled on the pages of my bird book. My journal described the details of seeing each new species and the excitement of exploring a wetland wilderness that was the largest freshwater marsh in North America.

I also learned to play soccer, drink high-test Canadian beer, and cut cards with the crew to avoid washing dishes after meals.

Several times, I met expert waterfowl biologists who came to visit, and they helped forge my destiny.

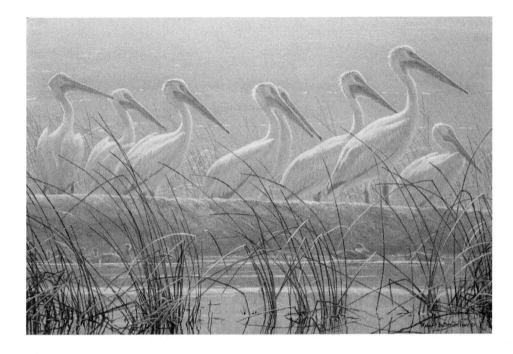

Bounty of the Wetlands

Surveys 2 through 4

I choose days replete with sunshine to run my surveys every seven to ten days, returning full circle to my days when I learned about ducks at Delta (once again packing bird books, field guides, and a journal for personal thoughts and reflections). If there has been rain, I wait a day for the roads to dry. If I am tired, I stay home. I know I am happy because I am dribbling across the kitchen floor, pretending to shoot jump shots down the hallways at home.

I maintain a gentle pace of work. As I approach each pond, I have time to view the habitat before selecting a starting point from which to begin systematically counting each individual bird, mentally noting the species and how many are males or females.

I can only remember a few birds at a time, so I quickly write them down, anxious not to lose my place on the water. I continue around the pond, being careful not to count any birds twice.

I have time to admire the birds and observe their behavior. I gather the look and feel of each new species, compelled to make sketches in my notebook, something I have rarely done during past field studies. Then it's on to the next pond until I finish the circuit, sipping black coffee as I go.

When I had conducted bird studies before my transplant, my ultimate source of satisfaction was often the accomplishment of having collected data. But now, though the quest for field data gives me a professional purpose and identity, I'm more excited to simply feel the world begin to shift each time I look out the open window at a pond. I can't touch the birds, but somehow, they are touching me.

It's idle work and I have time to be distracted by the nature around me. Each trip is a dose of paradise.

As spring progresses, the prairie comes to life. With each trip, the landscape becomes greener—grain sprouting, alfalfa growing taller, and golden bean blooming brighter along the roadsides. I drift from pond to pond, happy to flow with the nature that surrounds me.

I doze in the warmth of my truck, blissfully unaware of the trouble ahead.

Survey 5

Ducks mill throughout the pond, filling my binoculars wherever I look. I have little time to record them on my data forms, because when I look down to write, I lose my spot on the water. If I keep counting, to stay in place and not count the same birds twice, I forget half of what I have seen. There are hundreds of birds, there are twelve more ponds, and I have three hours to count them all. I panic about recording all the data within the four hours of the survey—it is mind-rattling overload.

I count hastily, trying to write and drive at the same time between ponds. I am exhausted at the end, my notes a shamble of loose pages long adrift from my clipboard. Some wear boot marks, others mashed crumbs. Some numbers have been repeatedly crossed out, while others are blurred with coffee stains. I would have failed my former students for such shoddy note-taking.

Transcribing the results takes over an hour. I re-check the numbers of each species as well as the proportion of males and females. I tally the numbers for each pond and calculate a grand total for all the ponds. When I double-check and cross-reference the numbers, small errors persist even after repeated attempts to find them. I must find the mistakes; even small discrepancies in data are unacceptable to professional biologists.

Watching a flock of teal skitter across the pond in front of me, I realize I am being afflicted by my old nemesis, chemo brain. The more birds there are to count, the faster my mind fails under the stress. It is like my problems dialing the phone and counting scoops of coffee. Now my brain struggles to transfer what I have seen to my hand and the paper.

More birds, many more, will arrive with the peak of migration—this is the prairie pothole region, home to some of the densest waterfowl populations in the world. Considering how the number of birds has recently spiked, I will likely encounter a peak survey population of 4,000 to 5,000 birds. It is going to be an incredible spectacle.

I can never count them all.

I will have to quit. The study will be ruined, and it is too late to find anyone else. I have that queasy feeling when you've done something wrong that you'd like to hide but you know you'll have to admit to the truth.

Fear races through me. What will happen to me? If I lose the duck counts, I risk losing myself all over again.

★ ★ ★ ★ ★

My daughters rescue me, skipping classes to record the data while I count. If I must work alone, I use a tape recorder, my eyes never leaving the pond. I train myself to stay on task and become a faster observer.

The crisis passes, aided by the departure of many birds migrating farther north. A pattern of lower numbers settles in by early summer, and I travel the circuit of ponds alone.

Each survey again becomes a golden day. I have time to pause and capture the critical moments of splendor I see. There are more than birds, and far more than data.

After each survey, I walk the prairie, trying to remember the names of plants that I see: prairie crocus, scarlet mallow, pussy-toes. A blazing star, flourishing on the loosely tilled soil of a badger mound, strikes me with its frothy lavender flowers, and I must stoop to touch it and inhale its mint-like scent. I examine plants, bugs and stones maybe a hundred times a day, and each time I feel like the boy I once was exploring nature.

When I try to recall the flowering sequence of the prairie plants that have yet to bloom (keen to test my predictions), I am conscious of coming full circle, back to my days as a novice biologist in the field when my first observation of a new plant (or bird or tree) was a uniquely amazing experience. A big part of the thrill then was being able to properly identify the specimen to its counterpart in a field guide. But now I feel more than the satisfaction of matching a new species to a picture on a page. Each new encounter is a sparkling fixture of time and place.

I carry no watch and use my shadow as a sundial, gathering the land and sky around me. As I wander, feeling the touch of wind and sun, I finally capture a familiar sense of space, one simultaneously near and far, my thoughts seamless. My feet begin to place themselves automatically to avoid the gopher holes hidden in the grass.

I don my chest waders—for the first time in years—to measure summer water levels in the ponds. I glide along effortlessly, unbelievably buoyant. As I float along, I marvel at a body free of fatigue. I return with a sweep-net to scoop pondweeds and water bugs, eager to learn more about what fuels the birds living in the wetlands—and to feel so magically weightless.

I often stay, overlooking the marshes, until I see the first stars. Darkness is rising from the ground, the sun still glowing somewhere behind the westerly mountains.

Nature is my nirvana. It is divine.

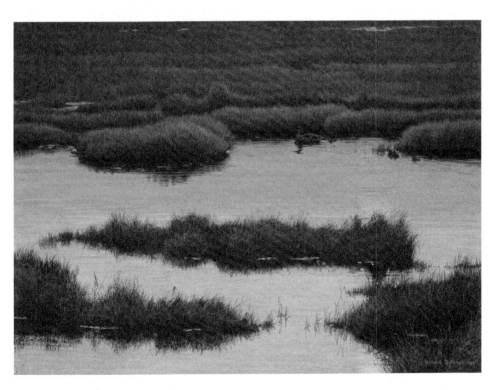

Mallard Family at Sunset

Chapter 23

Climbing My Mount Everest
(Chief Mountain)

My foot slips on a narrow ledge: in that split second,
as needles of fear pierce heart and temples, eternity
intersects with present time. Thought and action
are not different, and stone, air, ice, sun, fear, and self
are one.

–Peter Matthiessen, *The Snow Leopard*

I never expected to receive an invitation to climb a mountain.
Climbing peaks to the heavens is the realm of experts, brave
and intrepid mountaineers imbued with grit, a determination
nearing madness, and an unworldly degree of hardiness. You
need expertise in the use of ropes, cables, pitons, carabiners, and
other gadgets exclusive to the sport. I can barely tie a square
knot correctly—is it bottom over top, then top over bottom?
Right over left, then left over right?

The climb is not Mount Everest, but the request comes from
a man who has stood on that hallowed summit: Alan Hobson,
another survivor of Unit 57.

Alan guided the development of the exercise program I had
completed the previous year at the University of Calgary. He
is organizing a trip for climbers willing to donate money to

support further research into the benefits of exercise for cancer survivors. I would be along as proof of just how remarkable these benefits could be. Essentially, I would be the poster boy.

But can I hike for hours and climb to the top of a mountain? When was the last time I carried a pack with enough gear to weather rain and snow in the high country?

Despite my renewed body, I remain cautious about pushing myself. Walking around my study area after counting birds, I always stop to rest when my heart begins to pound in my ears. I have only truly tested my stamina once, fleeing across the prairie from a red Holstein bull that had escaped his paddock.

We will be climbing Chief Mountain, a massive square monolith of crumbling stone. The eastern face of the mountain rises 1,500 feet sharply above the prairie, easily dominating the front range of the Rockies in southwestern Alberta. Clearly visible from the outskirts of Lethbridge, the mountain is always a welcome sight when I near home, driving south from Calgary. I know it can be climbed from its southern backside without technical gear. I also know the way is unmarked, and that it is a treacherous hike for the weak or unprepared. I want to thank Alan for helping save my life. When he asks me to climb, I join the team: it is an offer I cannot refuse.

Our trek starts easily on an old logging road. Only a few hundred meters from the trailhead, we follow a narrow animal trail through thick scrub and wind-blasted trees that tug at my clothes and pack. The path leads down into a wet spruce forest and disappears where uprooted trees block our way. Only twenty minutes in and I am starting to lag the main group.

After scrambling over the tangle of dirt and deadfall, we hike hard uphill along the edge of a steep cut-bank where I must watch my feet to avoid tripping over the exposed roots and pitching into space. Eventually we enter the dense undergrowth of a thick forest, meandering downhill until we find an animal trail. It runs straight uphill through damp meadow grass to a destination hidden beyond the near horizon.

I lose sight of those ahead of me. My heart is pounding and I am puffing: if this were the old days, I would have been in the lead. Alan retrieves me, and I am relieved to see the rest of the group has asked for a short break

We wind uphill, single file, climbing through an uneven plain of house-sized rocks that ends at a mudslide. Only a few small plants grow in the plowed earth. Deer tracks are embedded in the dry mud, and I think what a slippery mess this would be if it rained later today.

Alan repeats a statement he has made several times: "Chief is the most actively eroding mountain I have ever climbed."

We travel in a loose group across the broken land. Even with a steady pace, it is a solid hour before we are across and together, counting off once again. We are still hiking diagonally away from the western flank of the mountain.

I want to ask how much farther we need to go before we stop hiking and start the ascent to the summit. I know I will go as far as I can, and will not quit until I am told I can rest. I remind myself of the test ride on the bike, but I must reach the top or I will let Alan down.

A broken field of jagged boulders blocks our way. Tilted at awkward angles, they shift precariously under my weight, so I move cautiously, testing each new foothold. I no longer have the strength and balance of my mountain-man days to leap naturally from rock to rock, as the others do ahead of me, so I sit and stretch a leg to the next boulder below me before reaching ahead to grab it. Serrated edges bite into my hand.

Another hour slides by as I scramble through the maze. Finally, after three strong hours of hiking across rough and busted terrain, we are ready to start our push to the summit.

Above us looms a long, steep slope of slippery, scree— broken rock fragments, rust-colored and purple-layered, that have bounced, rolled, and slid from the top. With each step, we will disturb the unstable debris. The true test of my endurance waits ahead.

I lean into the slope, trying to plant my feet, but I slide backwards, the loosely knit rocks slipping beneath my boots. I pick my way sideways, trying not to dislodge the bigger slabs above me. We spread out along the slope to avoid tumbling rocks on those below.

Occasionally I find a solid path of a few steps where I can rest before reversing my course to advance a few precious feet higher. Each switchback becomes shorter as I climb, the angle of the slope increasing steadily. I am soon stopping every few moments to gasp for breath and relieve the pain in my thighs. I never look back. I only look forward to my next step.

It had been easier to stumble along the hallways of Unit 57.

My legs are shaking two hours later when I reach a facade of crumbling rocks that blocks the final pitch to the summit. I follow the others into a hidden gap where we traverse a spiralling staircase of loose stones, looking for firm footing and solid places to place our hands. It's so narrow my face is touching rock. I pull myself up through the shadows, boosting myself higher until I emerge into daylight, nothing but blue sky in every direction. I slide my butt across to a flat patch of rocks, afraid to stand until I find my strength.

I had imagined a single peak, but instead there is a long ridge of cracked slabs no wider than a sidewalk. Gaps too wide to step across block the route to the highest elevation, so we climb down and up stacks of eroding rock to reach the summit where the natives have placed a cairn of animal skulls.

We hear thunder, so we hurry to descend. On the way back, I think of what the Blackfoot elder said to me the previous night following orientation. After he blessed our hike, I was asked to speak about my personal cancer journey. Hidden wounds surfaced quickly, and I faltered when recalling the unending days and nights of fear and loneliness, depression, and the devastation of fatigue. I had to stand down, tears blinding my eyes, choking on my words before I could talk about how I was gaining energy from nature.

As we disbanded, the chief approached me and said, "While I watched you talk, I said to myself, there is a real man. He is not afraid to show how much it hurts."

★ ★ ★ ★ ★

At the potluck supper held to celebrate the success of the day, Alan hands each of us a personally inscribed copy of his book, *Climb Back from Cancer.* Inside the front cover of my book, Alan wrote, "Today, you demonstrated again that you are a man of incredible strength, spirit, intelligence, and drive. I salute your bulldogged tenacity and triumphant climb back. Chief Mountain was but a shadow of your ascent and of your own inner Everest."

The words make me both humble and happy. I was no hero; I had just done what I could, thankful that tough nature had once again brought out the best in me.

Alan and I return to Chief Mountain the following spring to mark the route for the cancer recovery hike in July. The snow is knee-deep in the trees and we become lost in the fog. The summit is icy, and a wide crevasse blocks our way to its highest point.

Alan is confident that with a running start, we can jump across the chasm. It's easy for him to say; he has stood on the summit of the highest mountain on earth. My instructions are to fade to the left—while in midair—if I feel I am not going to reach the other side. That way I will fall fifty feet into a big drift of snow rather than plunge two thousand feet onto a massive pile of rocks. I follow Alan, steering far left upon lift-off, plunging waist-deep into the snow on the other side.

We sit on the summit, our boots swinging over the side, sharing mini-packs of cheese and peanut butter to fuel the long descent ahead. The brilliant sun warms our faces and the shining mountains make us reach for sunglasses. I lick a chunk of ice, freezing my tongue, thinking of how far I have come, always with nature as my guide.

Chapter 24
More Golden Days

Out here sights, sounds, and smells are explicit, everything is signal and nothing is noise; vistas appear framed in my mind's eye, and things happen that I have never seen before.

–Harry W. Greene, *Tracks and Shadows: Field Biology As Art*

Following those epic climbs of Chief Mountain, I continue to count waterfowl for another five years. I expand the study, ultimately counting birds every week from late March to mid-November: I wait for the ice to melt, and months later watch it creep across the ponds, hopeful of seeing tundra swans before freeze-up.

My immune system is strong, but because I still lack the normal level of neutrophils, I think about mosquitoes because some of them carry the West Nile virus. Lyme disease is spreading north, so I check myself for bulls-eye tick bites. I stop wandering through abandoned farm buildings collecting owl feathers because the mice that live there may have hantavirus. But these are minor issues that never disrupt my days. I don't have scientific proof, nor do I need it—I am healthier in body and mind when working in the field. I find sage to crush between my fingers so its sweetly pungent smell can remind me how blessed I am to be alive.

I rarely practice hardiness, but feel hardy nonetheless, so I disregard the earlier promise I made to myself by agreeing to count songbirds, busting my butt to rise hours before dawn. After racing between survey plots to beat the clock, I often lie down like a deer, leaving behind a bed of crushed grass before coffee lures me back to camp.

The long summer days that follow offer opportunities to rejoin the land of the living. I pitch bales, sit on dented tailgates drinking coffee, discuss the terrible price of cattle at the auction mart, and defend my position not to shoot gophers, coyotes, crows, and especially badgers. I occasionally take a puff off a passing cigarette.

I never tell Dr. Stewart about smoking (or the tattoo I'm planning to get) but during my annual checkup, I tell him again how much I love doing my field studies.

Then I say I believe I've graduated from the Centre and will no longer be seeing him for my annual cancer physical exam.

"I see," he says, smiling, "you don't think you have anything left to learn from us."

"I really have learned a lot, Dr. Stewart, but you can spend your time better now with someone else, although I doubt they will fax you their questions ahead of time, and keep a binder of notes and records like I've done," I say.

"Just wait here a moment," he replies, disappearing from the room. I sense he has just thought of something.

He returns carrying three very large binders overstuffed with papers, and a fourth about two-thirds full.

"These are *some* of your results, Pat. It would be nice if you could keep coming back for a couple more years."

I agree to postpone my self-proclaimed graduation for two years. After all, I like being part of his research.

★ ★ ★ ★ ★

It is my final day in the field. The rising sun is flat, long rays skating from the horizon. Gleaming shards of frost stick to the barbed wire; I don't know how they can form there.

The pond beside me is ice-tight, lit blue. The prairie rolls to the distant mountains that are becoming rosy as I drink the black coffee in the stained cap of my dad's battered thermos. I can almost hear him saying, "The first sip of the day is always the best."

There are no meaningful data to collect but I have come anyway, to reflect on my many days afield. Once, wondering just how many ducks I had counted during the seven-year study, I asked Katie to create a master spreadsheet to tally the total number of ducks from every survey (each year, she and Amy have collated my data and created the tables and figures I have needed for my annual reports—tasks I am unable to complete without errors).

How grand was the total? An astounding tally of 244,400 ducks, a quarter million. But despite the multitudes of birds, a sudden flare of iridescence would always turn my head, the red eye of a cinnamon teal would always unhinge my mind from the task at hand, and a glimpse of something new would always haul me over to the side of the road for a better view.

Now, I admire the few hardy mallards and Canada geese scrounging nearby for grain in a windswept patch of stubble. They will soon be gone, as the heavy snow that is forecast overnight will bury the last remnants of food.

I start the heater, despite being mindful of hardiness.

I will miss the anticipation and commitment to completing a day afield, and how I celebrate in the lee of a hill by the final pond, savoring the last of my snacks, replaying the most unusual or astonishing highlights of the day. Like when a pair of killdeer twisted and tumbled in mock broken-wing displays to lead me from their downy chicks, or when an anvil fell flat-out from the sky—a peregrine falcon crashing into a teal. Or when Amy and I watched a tail-less magpie flounder across the sky. These were the big moments of the day to be alive, and there had been many.

Even while driving in silence around the study area, I was never alone. The songs of meadowlarks always pierced the cab of my truck, even when I had the windows closed while speeding along the gravel roads. I was never far from the cries of hawks that circled above wherever I was, and there was always the dusty music of the wind through grass and sedge as I watched the birds working the ponds.

I am startled from these reminiscences by a snowy owl landing in a fallen tree. Black and brown feathers—a female descending the long way from the Arctic in search of a winter home.

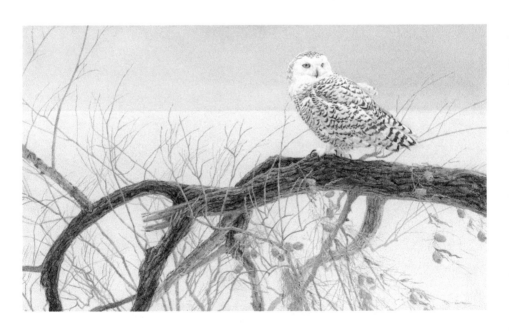

Fallen Willow - Snowy Owl

I see a magpie disappear over a hill and I begin to drive in that direction, running on nature, to see what lies ahead.

Epilogue

Reconnecting to nature, nearby and far, opens new doors to health, creativity and wonder. It is never too late.

–Richard Louv, *The Nature Principle*

I remain indelibly hitched to nature in all aspects of my life; usually the reins can be slack. And I am never far from that phenomenal day in the mall when the look of that tiger led me back to nature.

A few years ago, over a decade after my treatment, I was clinically diagnosed with a cognitive dissociative disorder. That was no surprise because at times I am still readily distracted, seeing things in complete isolation from their surroundings. And often with a single glance, fine textures and edges appear unbidden in everything I see.

Making coffee is still tricky, and I continue to have trouble with math.

But I can pursue long outings in nature, and during an August night, while drifting with orcas, I found I could also rely on a new source of hardiness.

I was floating with the pod, drifting ever farther from camp in the formidable current of the Johnstone Strait at the northern tip of Vancouver Island. I had no need to paddle, cruising along with the whales, trailing my hands in the cold steel-blue water, tasting the salt water (instead of pinching myself).

At times the sleek dorsal fin of the big female was so close that I thought if I leaned out far enough, I might touch her. Often, I could feel the mist of her breath settle on my bare neck and arms. Her wake was barely a ripple across the smooth, deep water.

I lost track of time—it was only when I saw the first stars of the night I realized I must turn back. The strong current and a stiff evening wind were now against me and there was no shore-bound light to guide me.

I steered in the long summer twilight for the mountain peak I knew was above my camp. I thought of all those I loved and had loved. And the many people who had enabled me to survive my days of emotional and physical crisis.

The thought of them kept me going through the choppiest waters of the darkest night I had ever been on the ocean. With them, I had become as resilient as the nature I so adore.

I paddled on. No distance too far.

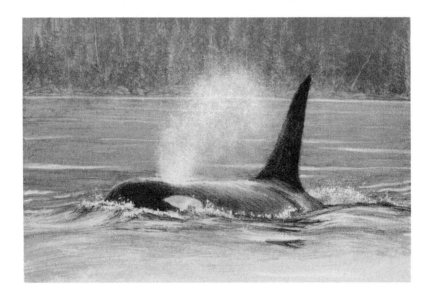

Fluid Power – Orca

Acknowledgments

My daughters, Katie and Amy, appear only briefly in this book. Without their steadfast love, encouragement and companionship, however, I would not have lived to share this story with you.

Many people were along on this journey, some for considerably longer than others. Their importance to my new life is significant, no matter how much time we spent together.

The love of my parents, Dorothy (Dottie) and Gerald (Jerry), was foremost during the uncertain years of watching, waiting, and treatment. I apologize for scaring you, Mom, with the chicken hawk talons you found in my jeans pockets, and for making you sit in the boat until dark while I fished for muskies, always promising you "just one more cast."

Dad, I am forever grateful to you for taking me along in the outdoors from the time I could barely walk. Pushing you in the boat through the muck of Crow Indian Marsh was easy to do, buoyed by those memories.

Susie Dietrich, Carol Coughlin, Richard Herzog, Michael Herzog, and Kathy Thomas, my sisters and brothers, were only a phone call away, and their visits always filled me with hope and encouragement, a situation that continues today. My nephews, Tyler and Jeff Thomas, threw me footballs and fastballs, and their dad Bob let me show him how to catch perch on a day when fishing was essential therapy.

To my special friends to whom I owe more than thanks: Richard Laing, for providing a home countless times over the years after my treatment, and for personal advice that made me laugh; Bob Machum, for getting me back in the field despite my protests, and for not complaining as I sought to overtake him as his parents' favorite son; Bill Berry, for keeping me safe as we traveled rivers and trails together when I was weak, and reliving with me our childhood memories of mischief; Shane Porter, for his determined care of me at the hospital and thereafter at both work and home, and for the thoughtfulness he showed my daughters; to Rita McMillan, for introducing me to Robert Bateman, fostering my love of art, and keeping this book alive as only a great friend can do; and to Lorna Marchi, for helping me love again.

I owe an incredible debt to the doctors, nurses, and staff at the Tom Baker Cancer Centre. Dr. James Russell gave me the confidence to accept the risk of my treatment with his thoughtful demeanor and expertise. Dr. Ahsan Chaudhry's smile and care meant the world to me throughout my stints on Unit 57, as did the demeanor of all the nurses and staff on the floor. A special thank you to Bolek Babiarz, who reminds me to this day to post my annual new-year photo for the hallway bulletin board.

Dr. Doug Stewart guided me with wisdom and concern during my countless appointments to the outpatient clinic. Karen Sabo, the nurse assigned to my case, met me there for several years. One time was particularly notable because when I arrived I announced, "I don't care what you tell me today, I'll be happy." Karen's response? "I don't know what kind of drugs you are on today, but go sit down and don't move until I get there."

Dr. Heather Hicks, you showed me how to put my life back together. I have never met anyone with your intuition on how to enable patients to heal themselves.

Dr. David Smith, Faculty of Kinesiology, University of Calgary, your program of exercise rebuilt my stamina and allowed me to return to my work with nature.

The high-powered professional expertise of these individuals and many others defeated my cancer, but it was the unfailing comfort of their human touch that allowed me to ultimately prosper, and their care is the true catalyst for this book.

Melissa Vicencio, Blood and Bone Marrow Transplant Clinic, Alberta Health Services–Cancer Care, thank you for responding to all my requests for current information on my procedure.

Laura Herzog, a cancer survivor, encouraged me to write with more emotion so that the story has life. I owe her a turtle.

Shauna McRae was a driving force throughout the two years I worked on this book. She patiently read several drafts, offering significant insight along the way, and helped me maintain my belief that my story was worth telling.

Wendy Fox and Louise Prud'homme provided thoughtful reviews of early drafts of the manuscript. Marva Blackmore, with support from Gerry Barnum, The Learning Centre, Parksville, B.C., began the editing process, and Mariah Carlsen pushed the process forward. Gayle Berry thoughtfully reviewed a near-final draft. But it was the personal insight, expertise and kind understanding of Jen Groundwater that allowed me to finally let this book go to print.

Amy De Nat ably guided me through the self-publishing process at *FriesenPress*. I thank her for her patience in answering my many questions.

Robert Bateman, a fine and generous man, allowed me to use his paintings. They are remarkable portrayals of my love for nature, and my story would be much less without them.

Thank you, everyone.

Grateful acknowledgement is made to the following for permission to reprint previously published material:

Credit: Copyright ©2010 George Schaller, from *A Naturalist and Other Beasts*. Reprinted by permission of Counterpoint.

Excerpt(s) from LAST BREATH: THE LIMITS OF ADVENTURE by Peter Stark, ©2001 by Peter Stark. Used by permission of Ballantine Books, an imprint of Random House, a division of Penguin Random House LLC. All rights reserved.

Excerpt(s) from AT THE WILL OF THE BODY by Arthur W. Frank. Copyright ©1991 by Arthur W. Frank and Catherine E. Foote. Used by permission of Houghton Mifflin Harcourt Publishing Company. All rights reserved.

Excerpt(s) from WHY BUFFALO DANCE by Susan Chernak McElroy, ©2006 by Susan Chernak McElroy. Used by permission of The New World Library. All rights reserved.

From A SAND COUNTY ALMANAC by Aldo Leopold, ©1949 by Aldo Leopold. Used by permission of Oxford University Press. All rights reserved.

From A MEMOIR OF LIVING AND ALMOST DYING by Wayson Choy, ©2010 by Wayson Choy. Used by permission of Anchor Canada. All rights reserved.

From A WALK IN THE WOODS by Bill Bryson, ©1998 by Bill Bryson. Used by permission of Doubleday Books, an imprint of Random House, a division of Penguin Random House LLC. All rights reserved.

References

Abbey, Edward. 1968. *Desert Solitaire.* Ballantine Books: New York, NY.

——————. 1982. *Down the River.* E. P. Dutton, Inc.: New York, NY.

Brenders, Carl. 2007. *Pride of Place – The Art of Carl Benders.* Langford Press: Narborough, Norfolk, United Kingdom.

Bryson, Bill. 1998. *A Walk in the Woods: Rediscovering America on the Appalachian Trail.* Doubleday Canada, Toronto, Canada.

Carlson, Linda E. and Michael Speca. 2010. *Mindfulness-Based Cancer Recovery: A Step-by-Step MBSR Approach to Help You Cope with Treatment and Reclaim Your Life.* New Harbinger Publications Inc. Oakland, CA.

Choy, Wayson. 2010. *A Memoir of Living and Almost Dying.* Anchor Canada: Toronto, ON, Canada.

Collins, Jim. 2001. *Good to Great: Why Some Companies Make The Leap . . . And Others Don't.* HarperCollins Publisher: New York, NY.

Frank, Arthur W. 2002. *At the Will of the Body: Reflections on Illness.* Mariner Books: New York, NY.

Greene, Harry W. 2013. *Tracks and Shadows: Field Biology as Art.* University of California Press: Berkeley, CA.

Gonzales, Laurence. 2003. *Deep Survival: Who Lives, Who Dies, and Why.* W. W. Norton and Company, Inc.: New York, NY.

Hobson, Alan. 2004. *Climb Back from Cancer.* Climb Back Inc.: Canmore, AB, Canada.

Leopold, Aldo. 1949. *A Sand County Almanac.* Oxford University Press, Inc.: New York, NY.

Louv, Richard. 2012. *The Nature Principle: Reconnecting with Life in a Virtual Age.* Algonquin Books: Chapel Hill, NC.

Matthiessen, Peter. 1978. *The Snow Leopard.* Viking Press: New York, NY.

McElroy, Susan Chernak. 2006. *Why Buffalo Dance: Animal and Wilderness Meditations Through The Seasons*. New World Library, Novato, CA.

Muir, John. 2009. The Writings of John Muir: The Story of My Boyhood and Youth. General Books LLC: Memphis, TN.

Park, Sooyong and John Vaillant. 2015. *Great Soul of Siberia: Passion, Obsession, and One Man's Quest for the World's Most Elusive Tiger*. Greystone Books: Vancouver, BC, Canada.

Roberts, Robin. 2014. *Everybody's Got Something*. Grand Central Publishing: New York, NY.

Schaller, George. 2010. *A Naturalist and Other Beasts: Tales from a Life in the Field*. Sierra Club Books: San Francisco, CA.

Selhub, Eva. M. and Alan C. Logan. 2012. *Your Brain on Nature*. HarperCollins Publishers Ltd.: Toronto, ON, Canada.

Stark, Peter. 2001. *Last Breath: The Limits of Adventure*. Ballantine Books: New York, NY.

Vaillant, John. 2010. *The Tiger: A True Story of Vengeance and Survival*. Vintage Canada, a Division of Random House of Canada Limited. Toronto, Canada.

Selected Bibliography

Abram, David. 1996. *The Spell of the Sensuous*. Pantheon Books: New York, NY.

Bateman, Robert. 2002. *Birds*. Penguin Books Canada: Toronto, ON, Canada.

——————— .2002. *Thinking Like A Mountain*. Penguin Books Canada: Toronto, ON, Canada.

———————. 2010. *New Works*. Greystone Books: Vancouver, BC, Canada.

Buzzell, Linda (ed.) and Craig Chalquist. 2009. *Ecotherapy: Healing with Nature in Mind*. Counterpoint Press: Berkeley, CA.

Clegg, Ellen. 2009. *Chemobrain: How Cancer Therapies Can Affect Your Mind*. Prometheus Books: Amherst, NY.

Cohen, Richard M. 2004. *Blindsided: Lifting A Life Above Illness: A Memoir*. HarperCollins Publisher: New York, NY.

Fisher, Karen. 2006. *A Sudden Country*. Random House: New York, NY.

Frank, Arthur W. 2013. *The Wounded Storyteller: Body, Illness, and Ethics*. University of Chicago Press.: Chicago, IL.

Henderson, Bill. 2014. *Cathedral: An Illness and Healing*. Pushcart Press: Wainscott, NY.

Herriot, Trevor. Frank, 2009. *Grass, Sky, Song*. HarperCollins Publisher Ltd: Toronto, ON, Canada.

Hoagland, Edward. 1999. *Tigers and Ice: Reflections on nature and Life*. The Lyons Press: New York, NY.

Hobson, Alan. 1999. *From Everest to Enlightenment: An Adventure of the Soul*. Climb Back Inc: Canmore, AB.

Hochbaum, H. Albert. 1973. *To Ride the Wind*. Richard Bonnycastle: Toronto, ON, Canada.

Holdstock, Pauline. 2015. *The Hunter and the Wild Girl*. Goose Lane Editions: Fredericton, NB, Canada.

Jordan, Martin. 2014. *Nature and Therapy: Understanding Counselling and Psychotherapy in Outdoor Spaces.* Routledge: Hove, East Sussex, UK.

———————— and Joe Hinds. 2016. *Ecotherapy: Theory, Research and Practice.* Palgrave Macmillan. New York, NY.

Keller, Shelli. 2013. *Improving Cognitive Function After Cancer.* CreateSpace Independent Publishing Platform (1870). ASIN: B01FYIDEMI.

Krakauer, Jon. 1996. *Into the Wild.* Anchor Books: New York, NY.

Lionsberger, John. 2007. *Renewal in the Wilderness: A Spiritual Guide to Connecting with God in the Natural World.* SkyLights Path Publishing: Woodstock, VT.

Lorbiecki, Marybeth. 1999. *Aldo Leopold: A Fierce Green Fire.* Oxford University Press: New York, NY.

Macdonald, Helen. 2015. *H is for Hawk.* Penguin Books Canada: Toronto, ON, Canada.

Matthiessen, Peter and McKay Jenkins (ed.). 1999. *The Peter Matthiessen Reader.* Vintage Books: New York, NY.

May, Gerald G. 2006. *The Wisdom of Wilderness.* HarperCollins Publisher: New York, NY.

Millard, Candice. 2005. *The River of Doubt: Theodore Roosevelt's Darkest Journey.* Broadway Books: New York, NY.

Newby, Eric. 1958. *A Short Walk in the Hindu Kush.* Penguin Books Ltd.: Harmondsworth, Middlesex, England.

Olson, Sigurd F. 1976. *Reflections from the North Country.* University of Minnesota Press: Minneapolis, MN.

Quammen, David. 2003. *Monster of God: The Man-Eating Predator in the Jungles of History and the Mind.* W. W. Norton and Company: New York, NY.

Roberts, David (ed.). 2000. *Points Unknown: A Century of Great Exploration.* W. W. Norton and Company: New York, NY.

Silver, Julie. 2003. *What Helped Get Me Through: Cancer Survivors Share Wisdom and Hope.* American Cancer Society: Atlanta, GA.

Silverman, Dan and Idelle Davidson. 2009. *Your Brain After Chemo.* Da Capo Press: Cambridge MA.

Simon, David. 1999. *Return to Wholeness: Embracing Body, Mind and Spirit in the Face of Cancer.* John Wiley and Sons: Hoboken, NJ.

Stewart, Christopher. 2013. *Jungleland: A Mysterious Lost City, a WWII Spy, and a True Story of Deadly Adventure.* HarperCollins Publisher: New York, NY.

Stolzenburg, William. 2008. *Where The Wild Things Were*. Bloomsbury USA: New York, NY.

Thich Nhat Hanh. 1991. *Peace Is Every Step: The Path of Mindfulness in Everyday Life*. Bantam Books: New York, NY.

Wheeler, Patricia R. 2013. *Cancer: How to Make Survival Worth Living: Coping with Long Term Effects of Cancer Treatment*. CreateSpace Independent Publishing Platform (1870). ASIN: B01FKTJYYI.

Williams, Terry Tempest. 1991. *Refuge: An Unnatural History of Family and Place*. Vintage Books: New York, NY.

Young, Jon. 2013. *What the Robin Knows: How Birds Reveal the Secrets of the Natural World*. Mariner Books, Houghton Mifflin Harcourt: New York, NY.

About the Author

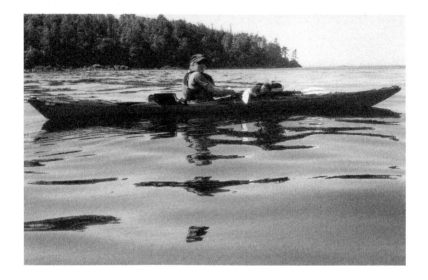

Photo: Ken Morgan

Pat Herzog was raised in Green Bay, WI, and earned a B.Sc. from the University of WI-Stevens Point and a M.Sc. from the University of Alberta in Edmonton. His career of forty-five years in wildlife conservation has included research and teaching with Ducks Unlimited (Canada), the School of Environmental Studies at Lethbridge College, The National University of Costa Rica, and the Department of the Environment, Water Resource Division, with the Government of Alberta. He is the father of three daughters and lives in Qualicum Beach, British Columbia. This is his first book.

CPSIA information can be obtained
at www.ICGtesting.com
Printed in the USA
LVOW05s0409080917
547786LV00008BA/14/P

9 781460 292723